RACHEL CATHAN is a writer fro introduced her to a part-time pu they had moved in together, aro and a little while after that – just made the exciting and terrifying ....y. ɪ ʌɪɪu ʋʜɪɪ, ʟɪke a growing number of couples today, well…not a lot happened.

Throughout the subsequent years of fertility investigations and failed treatments, Rachel kept a diary of her experiences, and it's from these first-hand encounters in the world of infertility and IVF that her first book, *336 Hours* has been adapted.

336 HOURS

RACHEL
CATHAN

SilverWood

Published in 2017 by SilverWood Books

SilverWood Books Ltd
14 Small Street, Bristol, BS1 1DE, United Kingdom
www.silverwoodbooks.co.uk

ISBN 978-1-78132-599-5 (paperback)
ISBN 978-1-78132-600-8 (ebook)

British Library Cataloguing in Publication Data
A CIP catalogue record for this book is available from the British Library

Page design and typesetting by SilverWood Books
Printed on responsibly sourced paper

For everyone who's done it, is gearing up for it,
or is stuck somewhere in the middle of it.
You may well be temporarily unhinged, but at least,
if nothing else, you are definitely not alone.

I've heard it said many times and by many people that there are few things harder in this life than having a baby. I think I'm inclined to agree.

Day One – Tuesday 31st January
The Final Countdown Begins

Symptoms: Insomnia, nausea, frequent urination, trapped wind and an inability to zip up even my 'Really Fat Day' jeans. This would be wonderfully encouraging if today were the last day of my two-week wait and our embryos were actually in my body right now. But, as it is, this is only day one of the fourteen-day torture, and so our embryos (if, indeed, we have made any) are still in a laboratory more than twenty miles away.

Hours until testing: 336
Waking hours until testing: 224
Predicted odds on this working: 5/10

10.00am

Okay, so here we go again.

Hello madness, hello fear, hello delusion and despair and sanity-shattering self-doubt.

Welcome all of my old enemies, won't you step inside and make yourselves at home, for we all know you will not be leaving my side for the next three hundred and thirty-six hours.

It is all so familiar to me by now, yet my intimacy with this process does little to relieve the tension. Rather, it reminds me that we are being swept ever nearer to the destination we have washed up at twice before. Except that this time there will be no return ticket; we will simply be staying shipwrecked on our desert island for two forever more. Or so we have agreed – in theory.

I wish I wasn't required to be awake for the next two weeks. It would be so much easier if someone could put me into stasis, like they do in science-fiction films, and simply wake me when this is all over.

But this is not a film, and there is no easy way to get through the minutes, hours and days that lie ahead.

And so the two of us sit, very quietly and very still, and we wait for my phone to ring.

It's hard to know whether it's a good or a bad sign when your embryologist still has not called by mid-morning. Is he saving us until last, so as to relish the joyous update that he's holding in store? Or is he simply putting us off, dreading the awkward moment when he must break the terrible news?

Already, I've received a call from Maria, the Spanish nurse from our fertility clinic, wanting a lengthy chat about what I've eaten and drunk in the last sixteen hours, the frequency, colour and duration of my toilet visits, and generally how I'm feeling 'in myself'.

I should have remembered this from our previous treatments: it's standard for a nurse to call first thing, just to make sure you're still alive and not developing any life-threatening complications following the egg-retrieval procedure.

The first time I had one of these conversations, I kept telling the nurse in question how nervous I was, hoping she'd take the hint, stop blathering on about water and urine and just tell me whether or not we had any embryos. But this time, I already knew that Maria wouldn't be the bearer of this news, so instead I took the opportunity to have a good old moan about the painful swelling in my stomach, the irony of my looking around four months pregnant, and the fact that every time I go for a wee, my swollen ovaries spasm in agony, confirming how happy they are that I've chosen to do this to them for a third time.

She thinks I'll pull through, Maria tells me in her sunny Mediterranean tones; my suffering sounds reassuringly normal to her.

What I want to tell her is that I already know I will pull through the *physical* side of this ordeal; it's the *psychological* challenge of the next two weeks that threatens to push me over the brink.

What to do with them, these three hundred and thirty-six thumb-twiddling, expanding and godforsaken hours of time? Unless I make a call to request that our broadband connection be terminated, I know how I'll be spending most of them: scouring the pages of the Internet for advice, hunting hungrily for the anecdotes of successful former IVF patients, whose stories might just keep me sane.

Of course, having dredged up these stories countless times before, I already know what they'll advise: stay busy…stay in bed for two weeks…go for long walks…keep your feet elevated…think positively…meditate…visualise…hold your breath and walk on eggshells…forget it all and carry on regardless.

And deep down I also know that these well-meaning soothsayers, these ghosts of the infertility journey, whose children's faces now adorn the IVF wall of fame, cannot foretell my destiny. They know what seemed to work for them, but they could never know what, if anything, will eventually work for me.

The reality is that I'm a lone traveller on this path, and there isn't another human on earth who can endure this test on my behalf.

Never mind wanting to be put into stasis for just the next two weeks; what I really want is for someone to knock me out and wake me only when I'm pregnant.

I'm not proud to admit it, but I've come to feel less and less interested in the weeks, months, years or possibly decades that stand between me and the moment when I'll look down at a positive pregnancy test.

Sometimes I wonder what I'd choose to do if I were told that this moment isn't lying in wait for me at any point in the future. Would I choose to hit the fast-forward button and skip through the next fifty or so years until I reached the day when it would all be over and I wouldn't need to contend with any of it anymore?

Some days I worry I actually would.

10.30am

Still no news from Steve, our embryologist. In the absence of his call, my husband (or DH as I tend to refer to him now – that's 'dear husband' in the world of online infertility forums where I now spend a good percentage of my life) has been busying himself with calls and emails from work, even though this is officially his day off.

As the hours have ominously ticked by, he has even resorted to collecting his discarded, dirty socks, which lie strewn in obscure places all over the flat, and loading them all into the washing machine.

Since I'm still bedbound from yesterday's egg-retrieval procedure, I have stopped even trying to find distractions for myself and have instead been actively visualising the separate petri dishes into which my seven microscopic eggs were placed yesterday afternoon, right before around 100,000 eager little sperm were added to each one.

In theory, IVF should be a sperm's idea of utopia: no exhausting Olympian swim up past the cervix, the uterus and the fallopian tubes with all the other riffraff in tow; this way it's more like a limo ride straight to the hotel door and then a brief scrum with the other 99,999 VIP members to determine who gets the keys to the honeymoon suite.

DH confessed to me earlier that he gave his little swimmers a quick pep talk before discharging them to the care of the embryologist yesterday morning, so we're hoping they were all crystal clear on the assignment they had chosen to accept. If for any reason DH's swimmers and my eggs have failed to get it on like Marvin Gaye advocated in the last twenty-four hours, then this mission will officially be over before it has even begun.

10.40am

I've finally graduated from the bed to the sofa, which makes me feel a little more respectable, even though I'm still in my pyjamas, tucked up under a blanket and toying with a cold slice of Marmite and cheese on toast (as if I could stomach even a grain of food before this call comes through).

Just as I was attempting to force down a tiny corner of crust, we received another heart-stopping call that turned out not to be the call from Steve. This time it was Jen, my younger sister, reminding me that I'm missing our grandma's ninetieth birthday celebrations tomorrow afternoon. I've feigned the symptoms of a fairly nondescript illness to get out of this event, mainly consisting of a dodgy stomach, since this is an acutely disruptive condition, but without requiring too much explanation or medical intervention.

Now I'm left feeling suitably guilt-ridden, for being both a horrible liar *and* a horrible granddaughter. But what can I do? Even if I didn't feel as though the inside of my stomach had been stapled to my groin, there is a familiar voice that is quick to break into the conversation and remind me that there's no way in hell I can attend.

'Well, what else am I expected to say?' this voice snarls in its defence.

Nothing, and I mean *nothing*, could be worse than attending a family gathering when you've been married for a suspiciously long period of time and have still failed to produce a single descendant. As far as my grandma's friends are concerned, I'm unsettling their worldview of human reproduction. Screw the fact that my grandma has made it to the ripe old age of ninety; all any of the meddlesome old crones will care about is: 'Why doesn't that granddaughter of hers have any children yet?' 'Is it that she *can't* have any children?' 'Or is it that…(oh, God, no, it's too unthinkable) is it that she doesn't *want* to have any children?'

To my face, the majority of them (those who can't yet use the early stages of dementia as a ticket to say what the hell they like) wouldn't actually voice these questions. Instead, they'd repeatedly ask me how long I've been married, assuming that if they ask enough times and force me to admit that it has been nearly FIVE years – yes, you heard that right, *five years* – then I'll eventually remember the names of all the children I've quite obviously given birth to since our wedding day. Failing that, they may choose to point out that I'm not getting any younger and that my sister (my *baby* sister) is already raising a five-year-old, a two-year-old and a one-year-old – and at the age of thirty-three!

If that doesn't persuade me to wheel out the kids I've been hiding from them all this time, then presumably nothing will.

I try, as always, to stifle this voice, to drown it out amongst the more pleasant, socially acceptable thoughts in my brain. But it speaks from the heart – from *my* blackened, bitter heart – and I cannot keep it at bay.

Gradually, it seems, the poisonous seed planted by infertility has been nurtured to maturity, in place of the baby in my belly, and has now grown into a hateful alter ego that threatens to consume my every waking moment.

The Fertile Myrtles of this world will NEVER understand how this feels.

Jen tried to convince me that my grandma's friends would never dream of asking the questions I so dread. But she is overestimating the tact and sensitivity of strangers by a pretty big margin if she believes this is the case.

I have learnt the hard way that people *can*, people *would* and, all too frequently, the bastards *do*.

My little sister and I have always been described (quite rightly) by other family members as being 'as different as chalk and cheese'.

Looking back upon our childhood, it seems to me that we travelled side by side as sisterly companions for such a brief period of time, before our paths forever diverged, our lives becoming incomparable, and virtually incomprehensible to one another.

From time to time, I have tried to imagine our roles reversed, but I've never quite been able to picture *myself* with the big house, the fulfilling career and the well-rounded kids, and Jen with…well, with what I have.

She is a woman accustomed to hammering her life into the shape that she desires, and 'can't' is not an answer she's ever been prepared to accept. Infertility simply would not suit the powerhouse I know as my baby sister.

And I imagine that if my problems really *had* been foisted upon her, then she would've put me to shame with her unwavering ability to power through and to cope. Well, unless, of course, the helplessness caused by this invisible illness had driven her to death by spontaneous combustion instead.

Perhaps I am better suited to these cards I have been dealt after all. Although, of course, we can't be sure that they are not going to kill *me* yet.

11.05am

He (the virtual stranger who today holds my heart in the palm of his hand, also known as Steve the embryologist) has dialled my number at last – and (thank God, thank God, thank God) has called to deliver some relatively good news.

Five of our seven eggs have fertilised and are looking well. Steve told us we now just have to wait two days, as is customary, at which point he'll call us again to tell us how our embryos are faring on their third day of existence.

As we thanked him profusely and ended the call, DH and I smiled at one another and breathed an audible sigh of relief. But this relief is not accompanied by the excitement we felt during our first two IVF treatments. The trouble is that it was always fairly good news from the respective embryologists on those cycles as well, and yet things still found a way to turn to total crap in the thirteen days that followed.

But dwelling on our previous failures is no way to drum up a positive mental attitude now, is it? We both know by this stage that IVF is nothing but a series of ever-steepening hurdles, and so we really must force ourselves to pause and to celebrate the survival of this latest jump.

On a different, and far more trivial, subject, I am slightly concerned that I seem to have developed the most severe case of trapped wind, or rather what feels like a trapped hurricane, in my stomach. This does seem to be the unavoidable result of having people digging around in your ovaries with a sharp needle and then pumping yourself full of medication whose effects mimic early pregnancy symptoms. Around once every half hour I've found that I'm able to release the most restrained, politest of little trumps, when what I feel is needed is for someone to stick a pin in me and then leave me to spin off around the room like a rapidly deflating whoopee cushion. In the end, I've had no choice but to kneel on the bed on all fours while DH attempts to 'massage out' a decent fart by rubbing my lower back. So far, we've managed to coax out two feeble little parps and one corker that sounded as though one of us had stepped on a duck. That last one was so impressive that DH had to stand back and congratulate me with a round of applause.

I've read that some IVF patients would be having sex around this time. They'd be trying to, you know, 'connect' and normalise the process of making their baby as far as possible.

Well, not us.

In fact, given the two-man wind turbine we have today put into production, I wonder whether or not we'll ever have sex again. And I also wonder whether or not it's a worrying sign that right now I hardly give a toss either way.

11.00pm

So, twelve hours on from our phone conversation with Steve (twelve hours of doing nothing but staying curled up on the sofa and watching TV) and the only question running around my head on a loop is: will this work?

If I'm honest, the positive attitude I forcibly drilled into my head a few weeks ago is starting to waver. One minute I'm telling myself that lots of people get to experience success after multiple failures, and the next I'm sombrely accepting the inevitability of another negative result.

It's troubling at this stage in the game, when it's far too late to back out, to sense that you may not be able to cope if the outcome isn't the one you want. *Especially* when you're faced with the reality that, statistically, the outcome you don't want is the one you're most likely to get.

I just wish it didn't matter so much. I wish I knew that I could take these next two weeks in my stride, smile if we emerge on the other side with the promise of a baby and, if not, dust myself down, walk off and plough full steam ahead with the rest of my childless (or should I say child-*free*) existence. But I've stumbled and picked my way through the wreckage that lies in the wake of a failed IVF treatment twice before, and I'm pretty certain that there is no shortcut back to normal life.

I promised myself that in this final two-week wait things would be different. I swore I would not allow myself to fall victim to the traps that have ensnared me in the past: the worrying, the overthinking, the early pregnancy symptom-spotting, the soul-searching and the general distraction. This time, I told myself I would be tranquil, enduring, strong.

I see now that I was a fool to think such a state might be attainable.

Even in this first day, I can feel that an important strand in the fabric of my brain has worked itself loose, and over the next thirteen days I can now expect the entire ball of grey matter in my head to unravel.

I know it's happening because this afternoon I found myself thinking that we will probably be required to buy a dog at some point in the near future.

Practically speaking, it would not be the most sensible of ventures. For one thing, it's actually against the rules of our tenancy agreement to keep a dog in the small, two-bedroomed London flat we're currently renting. For another thing, I'm distinctly allergic to all dogs, quite scared of most of them, and tend to dislike the remainder for being needy, noisy and smelly (some might well wonder why I'm nevertheless so desperate to have a baby).

But I don't want a dog because it would fit in with or enrich our lives in any way. I'm just grimly acknowledging that it's something I'll most probably need to add to my to-do list for this year, like renewing our car insurance and cleaning the stubborn, hard-to-reach patch of floor beneath the bathtub.

If we can't have a baby, then we will obviously be obliged to buy a dog, and this dog will be tasked with one very important mission: saving me from myself. It will demand that my reclusive bones are dragged from the flat to take it for walks each day, it will look up at me adoringly, it will accompany us on holidays to the coast, and it will be my loyal companion whenever I visit friends with babies or small children or get forced to attend weddings, christenings or elderly relatives' birthdays.

In the next instant, to confirm the brain-unravelling I suspected, I find myself abandoning the imaginary life with a dog and picturing instead a laboratory in a neighbouring borough, where five little embryos, five early versions of DH and me, are anxious to begin their second day of existence. All we need is for just one of them to show the same enthusiasm for, let's say, the next two hundred and seventy days, and we could be holding the baby we always dreamed of before this year is out.

It's hard to prepare, simultaneously, for two such disparate futures. And as this very long first day finally draws to a close, there is only one thing I know for certain: attempting to make a baby in this way evokes a strong desire to be wrapped in cotton wool and put into stasis for at least the next two weeks.

It is not conducive to participating in any definition of life in the real world.

Day Two — Wednesday 1st February

Living Life in Decaf

Symptoms: The overwhelming urge to visit a McDonald's drive-through and order an Egg McMuffin with hash browns (which sadly does not feature on my current organic, fertility-boosting diet).

Hours until testing: 312

Waking hours until testing: 208

Predicted odds on this working: 5/10

10.45am

I'm feeling a little guilty. Having resisted the urge to visit the nearest McDonald's drive-through, I've instead eaten an entire packet of Jaffa cakes, and it's not even midday.

I think maybe I just need to feel like I'm rebelling a little. As of yesterday, my body is not responsible for the development of anything or anyone. I'm growing neither eggs nor a baby; for the next few days my body is officially back to being mine. There's a part of me that would like to smoke twenty cigarettes, devour five tubs of Ben & Jerry's ice cream and then slosh it all back with a bottle of rum. I guess all my naughty buttons must be somehow interconnected, and nudging just one of them causes the rest to flash invitingly on the control panel.

It's probably not that surprising when a person's naughty buttons have been as repressed as mine have.

With the help of the internet and one well-intentioned nutritionist, I have, over the last few years, become suspicious of virtually everything I put in my mouth. I've been programmed to believe that caffeine and alcohol are toxic poisons and that one sip of either could render DH's sperm paralysed and clumped in a dying puddle before it reaches the end of his pecker, and my ovaries shuddering to a premature halt – perhaps, if we're lucky, half-heartedly spewing out a shrivelled egg or two in their final death throes.

I was of course warned by the aforementioned nutritionist that it was futile comparing myself to the crack addicts, winos and cheeseburger-scoffing chain smokers who can be seen carting their litters of offspring up and down the streets outside our flat. Apparently, what I need to bear in mind is that everyone is different and whilst the years of abuse these thoughtless fuckers have wreaked upon their bodies have served only to make their reproductive systems all the more robust and determined to create another generation, a post-dinner cappuccino and After Eight mint for me could render my poor, fragile little body entirely unable to procreate.

If this is true, then I have to say I'd like to stick my head inside my own neck and scream 'What's the *matter* with you?' down at my reproductive organs. I mean, aren't every living creature's genes pre-programmed to prioritise their survival, to ensure that they are passed on to future generations? Just how have my genes managed to overcome this most primeval of urges? While everyone else's are going forth and multiplying, my genes are presumably sitting around in the lotus position having existential debates, muttering to one another that they just can't see the point of it all to be honest.

Why am *I* not programmed for survival?

And, more importantly, why should I have to feel wracked with guilt for craving just a little junk-food comfort at my hour of greatest need?

In the pursuit of broadening my horizons and taking an interest in the world beyond the contents of my ovaries, I've spent the last half hour flicking through a newspaper, and have just been reading about this year's preparations for the carnival in Brazil. Travelling to Rio to see it first-hand is a daydream DH and I have been idly contemplating since our early twenties but, as has so often been the case in our lives, we've just never quite got around to converting the fantasy into reality. And so this morning I've been trying to picture the two of us, in amongst the crowds and chaos, watching float after float of sparkly, scantily clad people pass us by. And as usual, when I imagine an activity that DH and I might enjoy as a ~~childless~~ childfree couple, I've been channelling every ounce of mental energy into hoping that the cosmos will never allow it to happen.

I look at DH sitting across from me, at the opposite end of our minuscule London living room, and I wonder what it is that *he* is hoping for these days. He has always been so hard to read.

As I watch him now, he appears to be engrossed in a daytime cookery show about how to bake the perfect pastry. But I think maybe he just likes to lose himself in anything that takes him away from the troubles in his life and, more specifically, his wife.

It's no wonder really that he feels the need to escape; I don't think I'm a very fun companion anymore. These days, my idea of letting my hair down and going completely wild is hearing DH ask if I would like a cup of tea, saying yes, hearing him ask what type of tea I would prefer, taking a long pause and then replying, my giddy heart racing in my chest,

'…NORMAL!'

Yep, no herbal, fennel, nettle or lemon nonsense for me on the days when these wild hedonistic impulses take a hold. Oh no, it's caffeine-fuelled PG Tips all the way. And in an extra-large mug so

I can really stick my fingers up and give my fertility a final 'farewell, fuck you and thanks for nothing' as I swig it back recklessly.

I don't think I'd mind being so incredibly dull if we actually had a baby to show for it.

All my many friends with babies have complained bitterly during their pregnancies that their husbands or boyfriends are out at the pub again while they're stuck at home, desperate to down a glass of wine, or simply revel in a brief window of time when they could unscrew their bump and eat, drink and do whatever they fancy without feeling guilt-ridden about the consequences.

'You should try a five-year pregnancy,' I've wanted to yell at them. 'A five-year pregnancy with no alcohol, no caffeine, no treats and STILL NO FUCKING DUE DATE!'

On a recent trawl of the Internet, I made the discovery that my present pregnancy status puts me comfortably at the top of the world's leader board, usurping even the Alpine Black Salamander, a creature native to the Swiss Alps which has the longest known gestational period in the animal kingdom, lasting anywhere up to thirty-eight months.

This means that the Alpine Black Salamander who threw away her condoms and started knocking back her folic acid supplements on the same night I did is now enrolling her two fully metamorphosed young at pre-school. And I'm still standing here waiting for a positive pregnancy test.

And talking to myself enviously about the pregnancy status of an obscure Swiss lizard, which even I can see might be a rather worrying sign.

1.30pm

At my insistence, DH and I have just stretched out side by side on the living-room floor and listened to a relaxation CD designed specifically as a companion for IVF. Of course, DH is sound asleep and has been contentedly snoring since the first panpipes chimed in. I, on the other hand, have arrived at the end of this hour-long session feeling angry, irritable and verging on violent.

I think what incenses me the most about all this holistic, complementary…HOGWASH is, at the heart of it all, the thinly veiled insinuation that if I don't comply with it one hundred per cent, with a glowing positivity emanating from my very core, then I'll have no one to blame but myself if this all goes tits up.

Confronted by failure, the response I hear from the supporters of everything holistic is that 'You blocked it; you couldn't really have opened yourself up to it. You have to *believe* it before you can see it. Maybe on some level you *wanted* it to fail?'

Needless to say, I was in a foul mood when DH awoke from his refreshing snooze, and after we had sniped at one another for a good ten minutes, he suggested, not for the first time, that I go out and get a proper job again so I have something more important to occupy my time.

The full-blown argument that ensued followed a predictable path: me rehashing every hapless twist and turn that has led me to my unemployed status, and DH presenting the undeniable truth about my situation, namely that a career would give me focus, purpose, self-esteem, distraction and, let's not forget, A MUCH NEEDED INCOME!

Did he seriously think I was unaware of these facts, I had screamed at him. Did he think I hadn't worked out the *real* reason why most of us need a job in our lives?

While I was still in work, I'd heard it said that one of the major drawbacks to having a busy career is that you never get the chance to stand back for a moment and objectively appraise your life and where you're heading. I would now have to argue that this is the most compelling reason for staying in full-time employment. Getting the opportunity to stand back and fully appraise your life and what you're doing with it is not, in my opinion, an activity that suits the human mind very well at all.

For me personally, having stood back and soaked up my ~~childless~~ childfree, jobless, penniless status, together with my dubious and dwindling future prospects, I have reached the conclusion that the best philosophy for me would be to work as hard as possible, keep my eyes down, collapse into bed each night exhausted and never look beyond tomorrow.

But, as DH is well aware, it just isn't that straightforward. He knows that when I left my job more than a year ago now, I had been backed into a corner, certain (as was everyone around me) that I must eradicate all possible sources of stress in my life if I was to have any hope of becoming a mother.

'But there are a million other jobs you could do – or at least apply for!' DH shouted at me, slamming his hand down on the kitchen counter and sending an open bag of Brazil nuts (*my* fertility-boosting, highly expensive, *organic* Brazil nuts) skittering across the floor.

Yes, I had explained to him for the hundredth time, but who in their right mind would take me on now? A woman with endless medical appointments stretching ahead of her? A woman who needs to take time off to attend these appointments, to recover from the procedures, and to deal with what must by now be borderline clinical depression? A woman who, in the very best case scenario, would be making an application for maternity leave almost as soon as she stepped through the door?

DH (ever the rationalist) had then suggested that we could take a break from fertility treatment for the next year or so, giving me a chance to settle into a new job before things descended into craziness again.

It was at around this point in the conversation when I think I might've slightly (okay, *completely*) lost it. I mean, I'm *thirty-fucking-five*, for fuck's sake! My eggs are already half-knackered and I think we can all safely agree that they ain't likely to improve with age! If having children is the most important thing in the world to us, then time is of the essence. We *must* prioritise this mission above all else, even if it makes us penniless and miserable in the process. Surely he can see that…can't he?

It seems that he can't, and I could kill him right now, I honestly could. The more he says these things to me, the more I feel us drifting apart, the distance between us widening with each and every rational and logical suggestion he makes. I feel I'm shouting across the void to a total stranger, someone who couldn't possibly have accompanied me throughout each and every test and investigation of the last five years.

And when he takes on the role of this logical, somewhat callous stranger, I realise, suddenly, that it is just me against my infertile body, me against Mother Nature, me against the world.

At moments like this, my husband makes it very clear to me that I am truly on my own.

2.00pm

DH has gone out for a walk (for a break) and, while he said that he was happy for me to tag along (as he was running out the door), it was pretty clear that he wanted his offer to be declined.

Damn my body for forcing us into this dingy, depressing cul-de-sac.

We were different people five years ago, and our marriage felt stronger than so many others that I now see continuing happily all around us.

But everything has its breaking point and, as we approach the fifth anniversary of trying to conceive our baby, it seems we are being driven dangerously close to ours.

Why couldn't I just have fallen pregnant as soon as I handed in my notice, just like everyone said I would? Why couldn't all those office gossips and would-be doctors have been right for once?

I remember my work colleague Sarah being convinced that my fertility troubles would be instantly forgotten upon the arrival of my P45. She told me how positive it was that I could at last 'forget about work and focus *all* of my energy on getting pregnant'.

Ooooh, crap, I remember groaning inwardly at the time. I hope that's not what I think I'm doing; I hope that's not what my *body* suspects I've got in mind. Because something I've come to understand very clearly is that the human womb is much like the old-fashioned kitchen kettle, i.e. it will stubbornly refuse to cook anything while everyone is pacing around, holding their breath and watching it like hawks.

Everyone knows that the only way to get pregnant is to stop trying so hard, forget about baby-making and focus on something (ANYTHING!) else.

And similarly, everyone knows that as soon as you 'give up' on the idea of having a baby and buy a round-the-world plane ticket, your body will be lying in wait for you, ready to surreptitiously roll out one of the many embryos it's been storing all these years in a little pouch behind your spleen, and slip it into your uterus just as you touch down in Kuala Lumpur.

I can't help but wonder how this theory that your body will only ever work in direct opposition to your desires applies to other situations in life. Suppose one of my many 'new mum' friends wants to lose all the baby weight she's gained throughout her pregnancy and is finding that no matter what she does it just won't seem to budge. Should I advise her to relax, stick her feet up, stuff herself with Krispy Kreme doughnuts and then be happily surprised when she wakes up one day, when she's 'least expecting it', looking just like Nicole Scherzinger's long-lost twin?

I wish somebody could tell me what to do to get pregnant. Maybe if I were to eat only pineapple cores for the next six months? Or sleep in a mud-mask of pureed pine nuts and panda poo for a year? Or walk around dressed as a giant satsuma for the rest of my life (because, you know, orange is the, er, 'colour' of fertility)?

You name it, I would do it – if only I knew it would work.

5.15pm

So, DH returned from his walk and, in spite of the fact that we are still barely on speaking terms, we agreed that we would take a stroll through the town and find somewhere to go for a 'relaxed' late lunch.

What we hadn't anticipated when we left the flat just after three o'clock was that we were actually signing up to attend the daily school collection parade, featuring every young yummy mummy in our postcode.

Why must my path in life be strewn with these smug, fertile bitches? Every corner I turn I seem to be confronted by one of them standing there wrestling with a pushchair, shouting at a toddler or visibly feeling sorry for herself because she's so fucking exhausted.

The women who screeched up at the primary school gates at the end of our road in their 4x4s today were no exception, and they reminded me of the co-workers I grew to hate so very passionately in my last job. They were always the ones who had it all and yet wanted to be held up as martyrs and lavished with sympathy; the ones who believed that, because both their personal and professional ambitions had been realised simultaneously, they were now going to require at least one day off a month, preferably in a luxury spa, just to get over the excitement of it all.

Sometimes, casting an eye around my office, I had to laugh at just how easy other women made it look, casually slotting in one pregnancy after another around job promotions, house moves, enjoyable holidays and fulfilling social lives. They had no idea what they were missing out on, had they? My unique approach to motherhood that threatened to drive you into a straightjacket before you got within a fifty-mile radius of a positive pregnancy test.

Neither DH nor I acknowledged the horror of the yummy-mummy spectacle we were witnessing, but DH physically flinched on my behalf as we were forced to dawdle along behind the world's best-behaved brother and sister, each holding their mother's hand as they skipped along at her side and asked her eagerly: 'Mummy, Mummy, can we make that special pizza again for tea? Please, please can we?'

I wonder how resentful these encounters leave DH feeling (towards these perfect happy families, the world, or perhaps only me) that he now spends such a large portion of life feeling so ridiculously uncomfortable.

Returning home after a tense lunch involving undercooked paninis and cursory conversation, DH eagerly took solace in his ever-growing inbox of work emails, while I settled down in front of some mind-numbing docusoap on TV.

Now, sipping my third (scandalous) cup of caffeine-fuelled tea of the day, I'm starting to realise I might need another human to talk to about all this; someone other than DH, that is; someone who isn't neck-deep and drowning in this terrible crap just like I am.

In the beginning, there were plenty of other humans to choose from, because I was determined to be upfront and frank about the fertility marathon we were running. And that was probably because I honestly believed we were nearing the last lap.

At this stage in our first IVF treatment, the text messages from friends were already rolling in: 'How are you feeling?' 'When will there be news?'

But we made the decision a long time ago now that we'd no longer share with anyone the details of our treatments or what our next steps might be. It was the right decision, I'm still convinced, but being right provides little comfort in the face of the loneliness I now feel.

6.30pm

Oh, good God. My mother has just called me from the comfort of her hotel room in Manchester to make sure I feel 'involved' in the birthday celebrations. And she's spent half an hour regaling me with the edited highlights of the ninetieth birthday bash, providing a detailed report on the physical and mental deteriorations of my grandma and her friends since the last time she saw them. She added that she'd lost count of the times she's had to yell at people with hearing aids in the last few hours that, no, her eldest daughter really doesn't have a baby yet.

Jesus. I mean, I can understand why elderly people keep asking this question; they just want something 'nice' to talk about, something that doesn't revolve around illnesses and symptoms and whose funeral they attended last week.

It's just a shame that I'd far rather participate in an hour-long chinwag about bunions, colostomy bags and their rapidly impending mortality than a five-minute natter about my mysteriously absent babies.

Mum concluded her update by telling me, no doubt prompted by the enquiries she's received on my behalf today, that she totally understands why I stayed at home this time (she doesn't, but this probably *does* still count as progress) and that she 'happened to come across' a fascinating article on surrogacy amongst the hotel lobby literature she was flicking through this afternoon. She proceeded to explain that, should it come to such a time when it's deemed necessary to recruit a surrogate to bring *our* child and *her* grandchild into the world, then she'd like me to know that she will be first in line for the job.

I can only be thankful that DH has never been in earshot when these offers have been made. Aside from the daytime chat-show nature of the proposed scenario, I know he already feels inept enough when both our mothers bring us food parcels and start cleaning the flat and tackling piles of ironing whenever they come round, without one of them taking it upon herself to actually grow our baby for us.

I understand where my mum is coming from, of course. This must remind her of the times she's had to watch me faff around whilst trying to grease a cake tin, or turn back a hem, or assemble flat-packed furniture. I guess you can just stand back and witness the mind-boggling incompetence for so long, but then you're forced to start thinking about who's going to be left picking up the pieces when it all goes wrong. To be fair, she's given me almost five years now, while she's stood patiently on the sidelines and let me have my go. But now, since neither of us is getting any younger, she knows it's time to stop buggering about, roll up her sleeves, and send in someone who knows how to get this task done.

It *is* incredibly kind of her to offer, I suppose, and especially after the heartache she herself has been through over the last couple of years. And so I forced myself to count to ten, thank her for her generosity, and not point out the biological unlikelihood of a woman in her sixties actually being able to fulfil the proposition.

If I'm honest, I *am* grateful for her unwavering support. And if I'm being *really* honest, I have to admit that it's hard (okay, verging on impossible) for other people to ever say or do the right thing by me these days.

10.30pm

Since I can barely keep my eyes open, I've decided to head up to bed early, leaving DH watching something on television about robots and futuristic gadgets that might be invented in the next fifty years.

I wish I could find the words to make everything okay again after our earlier argument, but quite frankly I just don't have the energy for a rematch, which is pretty much guaranteed when two people, who still wholeheartedly believe they are right, attempt to reconcile after a disagreement (or, in other words, offer the other person the opportunity to apologise unreservedly for their stupidity).

We both know ourselves and each other well enough by now to realise that there is nothing to be gained by this sort of exercise.

Tomorrow DH must return to work, leaving me to await the next call from Steve, when he'll tell me how our five embryos are progressing, what grades they've been awarded in their first evaluation, and what their likely prospects are if we transfer a couple of them tomorrow or wait another couple of days in a bid to determine (as my dad memorably joked during our first IVF cycle, just shortly before he died) which one might be eligible for the Young Embryo of the Year award.

Ah, my dad. I often find myself wondering what he would have to say about our current predicament. I imagine most women probably try to avoid fatherly/daughterly conversations about their attempts to conceive a baby, but my dad was always one of those pragmatic, unshockable types; the kind who'd trek for miles through remote Spanish villages to mime 'sanitary towel' at non-English speaking shopkeepers because you'd unexpectedly got your first period in the middle of a summer holiday; the kind who wouldn't bat an eyelid at talk of fertility investigations and the horrors of IVF.

The kind of dad I know DH will be, as it happens. Well, *would* be. *Might* be. One day.

If my dad *were* here now, just like DH, I know he would still be optimistic about our chances. Men: for some reason, positivity in the face of ~~childlessness~~ childfree...er...ness just seems to be hard-wired into them.

But a disheartening reality of both the 'day three' and 'day five' transfer options is the fact that we've probably produced hundreds of embryos before now (around thirty through our previous fertility treatments and God knows how many through our natural cycles) and, for reasons we may never understand, not one of them has been strong enough to become even a positive pregnancy test.

It's hard for me, following such a catalogue of failures, to believe that one of these five really will be able to break the mould. But, hard as it may be, I know that for the next three hundred and twelve hours, I will be clinging on oh-so-very-tightly to the hope that one of them might just prove me wrong.

Day Three – Thursday 2nd February

Groundhog Day... Again

Symptoms: Indescribable tiredness that's starting to feel like a hang-over (caused by the backlog of sleepless nights I've had recently), extreme clumsiness, a stubbed toe and a sore head (as a direct result of the clumsiness), and that persistent stomach-stapled-to-groin feeling that I've had since day one.

Hours until testing: 288

Waking hours until testing: 192

Predicted odds on this working: 6/10

9.05am

Sitting in front of the morning news with a bowl of organic porridge earlier, I thought it somehow appropriate that I should find myself in the middle of yet another IVF treatment while, across the pond in America, celebrations would be taking place in honour of Groundhog Day.

I've many times heard IVF described as a roller coaster ride, an up-and-down blur of breathtaking highs and death-defying lows, but as time has gone on, I'm more inclined to think of it as a monotonous kind of Ferris wheel. There's an eerie feeling of déjà vu as we whir around and around, passing the same old landmarks, before creaking to a standstill alongside the very tops of the poplar trees. Here we sit, suspended, twisting in the wind, staring out towards the horizon because we're too damned scared to look down. And then we inch slowly downwards, grinding to a temporary halt during every step of our descent, until eventually the ground is in sight and we're wondering if it might finally be our turn to get off or if we're going to be forgotten, left to spin around and around for all eternity, while everyone else hops on and off all around us.

The phone on my bedside table leapt into life at 8.15am this morning, striking fear into my heart that this might be one of his first calls of the day. That is, one of the calls that Steve has to quickly tick off his to-do list so that he can then start to breathe once again and get on with the more enjoyable side of his job.

I wanted to take my default position, to wimp out and throw the phone to DH as if it were on fire. This is, after all, the bargain we have reached: I deal with the toe-curling procedures; he deals with the nerve-racking phone calls.

But since (as he's so eager to remind me) someone in our household has to go out to do an honest day's work, I was the only one available to receive the update.

It's good news, Steve said hurriedly. (Phew, phew, *phew* – thank you, embryos, thank you, Steve, THANK YOU, GOD!) Three of our five embryos are looking strong, with the remaining two possibly still developing, just a little more slowly. So with no standout winner just yet he'd like to culture them for a couple more days in the lab and aim for a blastocyst transfer on day five.

A blastocyst, even though it sounds like something you'd find orbiting around the solar system, or something a teenager might wake up to find erupting from the end of her nose, is actually the one thing that everyone hopes to achieve in this game.

But one thing that DH and I have learnt over the last couple of years is that assessing embryos is a complex task. And we have always found it disconcerting to watch the number of seemingly viable embryos decline as the days pass by. Initially, we had assumed that every embryo equals a baby, but sadly this is far from being the case. More often than not, we have learned, none of the embryos produced will equal a baby; if you're lucky, then one or two just might.

The final decision about when to have the embryos transferred is down to us, and part of me wanted to have two of them transferred today, mainly so that I'd never have to face up to what they're going to look like on day five. But then if we *had* gone ahead and transferred two of them today, I'd still have to face up to what the *remaining* embryos were going to look like on day five. If they had stopped developing, I know I'd be taking it as confirmation that the two we had transferred had stopped developing as well. Whereas, if the remainder continued developing into first-rate blastocysts, I'd be worrying that they were the *only* healthy ones in the batch and that we had selected the wrong two to be transferred today. Either way, I'd be left feeling certain that we had made the wrong decision, and so in the end I agreed to simply follow Steve's advice, and then I'll know that whatever happens, at least I'll always have somebody else to blame.

Ultimately, I guess either this thing's going to work or it isn't, and the intricacies of how we play out the next few days probably won't make a difference to the end result. And in any case, I can't dwell on this almighty mind-fuck right now, since it's time for me to drag my battered body to work. I use the term 'work' quite loosely in this instance, since I am only volunteering to help out at a local charity shop.

I'm aware that it can hardly be classed as the next rung on my career ladder and that it will never be an impressive update with which to regale my old work colleagues should I bump into them on the Tube. In fact, due to its voluntary nature, I can't even claim it's a means to put food on the table.

However, it *does* get me out of the flat, which is almost as important these days.

The small run-down shop on the corner of our road is managed by a militarily organised yet cheerful woman called Carol, with the help of a narrow-minded busybody called Sylvie, the latter of whom seems to work a random schedule that, six months on from my start date, I still haven't quite been able to fathom.

For the life of me I can't remember whose turn it is to open the shop today, but I hope to God it isn't Sylvie's. Although, as I pull on my hat, scarf and gloves to brace myself against the arctic conditions outside, it occurs to me that, with my brain in its current sieve-like state, I should probably just be hoping it isn't mine.

5.50pm

On my short walk to the shop earlier, I phoned DH to update him on how things are progressing over in the laboratory. As dutifully as always, he told me it all sounds very encouraging and he's looking forward to the embryo transfer on Saturday.

This leads me to conclude that either he no longer cares about the outcome and is just telling me what he thinks I need to hear, or he truly has become the master of optimism.

Either way, I wish I could borrow his 'everything will be okay' mantra, if only for an afternoon. Unfortunately, my brain appears to have been wired without the everything-will–be-okay chip. And besides, there is something significant that sets me apart from the majority of women in my situation. I've noticed that most other women feel happier when their embryos are removed from the sterile Petri dish in the lab and transferred to where they rightfully belong: their ready and waiting wombs. I, on the other hand, feel much happier while our embryos are being monitored in their artificial surroundings. In fact, I think our fundamental and fatal error in the past has been returning the embryos to my body. My real fear is that these painstakingly created embryos are about to be transported into the deadliest and most inhospitable of environments; one where their many might-have-been brothers and sisters have previously perished.

If it were possible to grow our babies in an incubator for the whole nine months, I know I'd feel so much more confident. Then DH and I could just drop in on them every day, stroke the outside of their incubators, read bedtime stories aloud to them and vocally nurture them, like flowers in a greenhouse, to full size.

Come to think of it, what the hell have these reproductive endocrinologists been playing at? The first IVF procedure was carried out more than thirty years ago – why aren't embryos being grown from scratch in an incubator by now?

I must remember to ask this important question, together with 'Why aren't female patients put into stasis for two weeks after the egg-retrieval procedure?' next time I see our consultant, Dr Rangan.

For the next couple of days, however, I must simply resort to those wonderful, failsafe traditions of 'looking after myself', 'thinking happy, positive thoughts' and 'keeping my fingers firmly crossed'.

So, as it transpired, when I turned the corner at the end of our road and peered between the mannequins in the front window of the shop, it was Sylvie's frizzy copper-red curls that I could immediately see bobbing around behind the till. 'Bloody typical,' I muttered to myself as I pushed through the heavy shop door. Even the faint glimpse of her worry-lined forehead was enough to make me seethe, and I couldn't imagine how I was going to survive four long, tedious hours in her company.

To make matters worse, I quickly discovered that she was in one of her infuriatingly chatty moods and insisted on revealing to me the minutia of the lives of her three grown-up daughters. By the time she'd finished, I'd learnt that Helen had two girls, Vivienne was seriously considering a boob job after breast-feeding her firstborn, and Yvonne had three boys, which Sylvie thought preposterous since she was the least sporty of the bunch.

'Of course, the boob job can't happen because Vivienne's expecting her second now anyway,' Sylvie concluded, as we sat unpacking the enormous bag of clothes and toys that had been left outside the shop door this morning.

'Of course,' I agreed, turning away to place a bedraggled-looking teddy bear in the shop window.

'I meant to ask you about your family,' Sylvie piped up a short while later, a quizzical expression on her face as she transparently wondered how best to phrase the nosey and personal question she was itching to ask.

My chest tightened and my heart began to pound as I braced myself for the painful intrusion.

'What about them?' I replied through gritted teeth, determined not to make the conversation any easier for her than she deserved.

'Well, I wondered if you and your husband had wanted any children or…if you were one of those couples who'd…decided not to have any.'

One. Of. Those. Couples. Well, fuck you, Sylvie! And fuck you threefold for using the past tense when the present would have been sufficiently cutting.

Finding myself on the receiving end of this comment was one of those crippling moments where I caught a brief glimpse of myself through the eyes of another; where I saw clearly that while I'd been busy battling on at the front line, everyone else, unbeknownst to me, had accepted that my battle had been fought, lost and forgotten a very long time ago.

The perfect retort to Sylvie's statement was, as ever, elusive;

her cruel words had left me winded and it was all I could do not to burst into tears and crumple in a heap on the shop floor.

'Well, not everyone gets everything they want in life,' I told her finally, acknowledging my mistake the instant the words had left my mouth. A fatal chink in my armour had unintentionally been revealed, and I knew Sylvie would now be whittling away at that weak spot for as long as I was trapped with her in this shop.

'Oh,' said Sylvie, fiddling nervously with the gold chain around her neck, 'I hope I haven't hit a nerve.'

She stood still, biting her lip for a moment, and I thought she was going to change the subject, but instead something must have persuaded her to plough full steam ahead.

'Terrible thing when a woman can't have a child,' she told me, 'terrible, terrible thing. But you know what? I'll bet that dear old dad of yours is watching over you right now. And I'll bet you any money he's going to send you a baby before this year is out.'

Oh, here we go; I should've known she'd be resorting to that old chestnut soon enough.

I don't know who made these fertility rules, or where I was on the day that everybody else sat down to learn about them, but there are a surprising number of people who'll tell you it's lucky (yes, lucky) when a family member dies, the idea being that the fertility gods operate some kind of 'one in, one out' policy, so that the untimely departure of someone close could actually pave the way for a new addition to be created.

It's hard to know which is worse sometimes: life throwing you the lemon that is infertility in the first place, or the utter bollocks people will spout at you when it happens.

I drew a deep breath in preparation to inform Sylvie that the fertility gods appeared not to have noticed my dad's absence; to ask her whether she thought I should rub out a few other family members just to make sure – maybe invite them round for a Sunday roast and then slip them a dose of cyanide to see if that would boost our baby-making success rate at all.

But, luckily for me (or maybe for Sylvie), we were saved at that moment by an elderly and clearly infirm woman trying to ramrod her way through the shop door with the front half of her Zimmer frame. I rushed forward to assist her, grateful for the distraction and glad, as always, for our shop's aged clientele. I treasure the fact that this job has brought me into contact with so many people who share my view that life is a stinking sack of shit, and who are as wonderfully reliable as I am in terms of never turning up pregnant. These are pretty much the only two qualities I look for in anyone I'm required to speak to these days.

A few hours later, on my way home from the shop, I decided to stop off at our local café for a cup of peppermint tea and a pleasure-free muesli bar (a glass or ten of wine would have felt somewhat more appropriate but I was buggered if I was going to let Sylvie scupper my organic, fertility-boosting plan at this late stage in the game).

It was 4.15pm by the time I got in there – safely past the height of yummy mummy lunch hour, which I long ago learned to avoid. (Christ, there are so many ludicrous restrictions and restraints on my life right now; it's as though I belong to some sort of underworld, filled with vampires, prostitutes and other infertiles, and it's only appropriate for me to venture out as dusk begins to fall and the good people of this world – the happy-clappy families – are heading home to a nice cup of cocoa by the hearth.)

I'd picked the ideal time for a solitary dining experience, as it turned out. Well, apart from a couple of teenagers, who sat stroking each other's cheeks, giggling, whispering sweet nothings and then snogging each other's faces off in the corner of the café.

As I consciously tried to block them out, gripping a scalding mug of tea for the illusion of warmth, I found myself feeling absurdly jealous. How lucky the little shits were, I thought to myself, to be sitting there, so intoxicated by the present moment, so insulated against the rest of the world, so blissfully ignorant of what life held in store for them further down the line.

I know I too have enjoyed that ignorance, felt those beautiful butterflies in the pit of my stomach…but it all seems like a memory from an earlier lifetime now.

I found myself wondering if it's too late for DH and me to resuscitate a sparkle of romance in our own relationship. But it was a fleeting fantasy, and one that I knew could never be realised.

Having had my eggs collected three days ago, I had to remind myself that I was hardly in any physical state to greet DH from the train station in suspenders, high heels and a rain mac – or for any sort of encounter more intense than holding hands.

I think I just need to face the harsh facts here: we are not loved-up teenagers any longer, and trying to make a baby in this way is calculated and clinical, and there's not a thing we can do to pretend otherwise.

And it's probably also time to admit that infertility has totally put the socks, crocs and bobbled nightcap on our sex life.

I can still clearly remember how horrified DH was at the start of this nightmare (all those many years ago), at the very prospect of subjecting ourselves to tests, investigations and discussions with complete strangers about this most intimate part of our lives.

Maybe he imagined that we'd be ushered through to a room, ordered to undress and then instructed to hop up on a table and get down and dirty in front of a panel of experts, so they could all take notes, and tell us exactly where they thought we were going wrong.

For some reason, DH still believes I've come to welcome all

this intrusion, to depend upon it even, and he has lodged regular complaints over the years about how fed up he is of pulling back the covers to our marital bed, only to find that another 'expert' with their contraptions, helpful suggestions and prohibitions appears to have moved in. He tells me I'm guilty of sweeping him aside, of scrambling over him to get my hands on whatever it is that's the latest craze and forgetting that he's still an integral half of this equation.

'Maybe *this* will be the thing that gets me pregnant!' I've been known to yell, clasping a packet of vitamins, herbs, supplements or lubricants and shaking them excitedly in DH's face.

'Well, I wish you both the best of luck,' he normally laughs, 'but I think it will be a first if the two of you *do* manage it on your own.'

Oh how incredibly lucky all those normal, fertile bitches are; the ones who just casually pounce on their partner one night and then two weeks later miss a period, take a test and scream out, 'Oh, honey, guess what? I think we're having a baby!'

Those normal, fertile bitches really have no fucking idea. And I cannot tell you how much I wish I had no fucking idea either. What I wouldn't give to erase from my mind all the interesting facts I've acquired about cervical mucus and what its varying colours and textures can tell me about the inner machinations of my reproductive organs. What I wouldn't give to get back some of the *time* I've spent fishing around in my own cervical mucus in order to pick up on the subtle clues my body might be trying to send me.

Of course, some people imagine that trying for a baby for five years must be a regular fuck-fest.

'Ooooh, you two must be at it like rabbits,' some of my friends with children have commented, before telling me how envious they feel, and how their offspring are so energy-sapping that they can barely muster the enthusiasm to do it once a month.

The truth, not that I often share this with them, is that infertility can destroy a sex life more ruthlessly than a fractious toddler ever could. It can reduce a couple to the most boring, mechanical of encounters, encounters where neither party is remotely in the mood, but where they know that they *must,* to at least be in with a shot in hell, and to avoid a situation where, two weeks later, they will only have themselves or each other to reprimand for not being pregnant once again.

At its most soul-destroying, it might even see one half of a couple breaking off mid-session to search for, unpack, prepare and insert a *litre* (because more modest quantities have proven ineffective in previous months) of sperm-friendly lubricant into her vagina. And as she does this, she will know that as foreplay goes, it's an activity which can only be marginally less erotic than interrupting the throes of passion to gouge out an ingrowing toenail. But, to his credit, her partner will try valiantly to pretend that he is somewhere more appealing and to maintain the level of interest required, not fully prepared, of course, for the fact that when he finally resumes his task, it will feel very much like sticking it to a tub of cold custard.

At least, I *imagine* this is the sorry state of affairs that people in this situation might find themselves experiencing. And probably right before they eventually arrive at the stage where they're too miserable and too dejected to even shag at all.

Ha! This really is the moment when infertility bursts through the ribbon at the finishing line, triumphantly goes to collect its golden cup and starts to run victory laps around the racetrack.

On the plus side, I suppose, there is also the occasional month when you can't help but rebel against it all a little; the odd month where you decide you're going to do it *when* and *how* you want to, and do it very deliberately in the wrong position at the wrong time of day and during the wrong time of the month.

I know I have found it surprisingly liberating after all this time to do it *without* lying there afterwards with my legs vertically propped against a wall, while DH and I conduct a verbal debrief on our latest effort, commenting to one another about what a 'good one' that was, how we're certain to have 'nailed it' that time and how we'd just like to see me *try* to avoid getting pregnant after that shag-a-thon.

But this freeing mindset has only been allowed to surface as I've come to the very end of my rope with the whole baby-making fiasco – and it's a mindset that, with the greatest determination in the world, I can only seem to sustain for the briefest snippet of time.

And we all know why that's the case.

As I flicked on the harsh strip light above our bathroom mirror this evening, I instantly understood why Sylvie had asked me if DH and I had decided never to have children. The reflection staring back at me looked at least one hundred and eighty years old. And post-menopausal.

Christ, I can almost *feel* the menopause, evil witch that she is, alive and breathing inside me tonight, can actually watch her staking her claim on my body through the beginnings of crow's feet around my eyes, the worry lines on my forehead and the grey hairs sprouting from my scalp. This is the easy terrain into which she'll sink her first poisonous little flags. But soon enough these little flags will start to multiply and spring up across my entire body, until one day soon she'll snatch away my very last vestige of youth and officially claim me as her own.

I try, just like every other ~~childless~~ childfree woman my age, to shake off this evil witch, to tell her I don't care for her right now. But she sits on my shoulder like a devil, her gnarled old hands bending my ear, whispering to me that if I want to be a mother then this month is better than next, today is better than tomorrow, and every period I have from here on in is another month lost to me and another gained for her – one month nearer to the day when she'll burst forth from beneath my skin where she's been lurking all along and reveal me to be a shrivelled and barren old hag.

Oh dear god! I need to sit down and have a cup of decaffeinated tea immediately. I need to plaster on some anti-aging cream, take some deep breaths, put things into perspective. I must at least attempt to resist this terror, to retain the steady, unwavering mantra that good things come to those who wait, and that these good things will undoubtedly happen in their own good time.

Oh God, *please* tell me I have at least a couple of decent eggs left in me to try to create our baby. Please tell me it isn't already too late…

10.30pm

Trying to forget my heart-stopping encounter with the bathroom mirror this evening, I've been curled up in bed, a pillow propped beneath my swollen stomach, watching a documentary about emperor penguins.

The temptation to rush into the living room and offload the details of my gruelling day onto DH as soon as he entered the flat this evening was overwhelming – but self-preservation prevailed.

I know that if I dared complain about my day, I would be asked to explain what could *possibly* be so stressful about spending four hours 'working' in an incredibly quiet charity shop situated less than two hundred yards from our flat. And, put on the spot like that, it would be hard for me to answer that question.

And so instead I kept it all in, asked DH about his day, and asked myself, as I often do, whether I think he will eventually leave me.

The most terrifying realisation, when I start following this train of thought, is the fact that I am a woman entirely out of options now. If DH were to be revealed as a serial gambler, a serial philanderer, or probably even a serial *killer*, I worry I'd just have to sigh, ruffle his hair as though he were a badly trained puppy, and go back to reading about the latest fertility breakthroughs on my iPad. Because how would I doggedly pursue my fertility treatment without a dutiful husband in tow? And how long would it take me to find a suitable replacement – someone who would love me enough to risk sacrificing his own future children, and to pay for my food and board and medical bills, *and* to accept nothing but celibacy and mental dysfunction in return? Many years, I'm guessing. Or, more likely, forever. Either way, I'd be menopausal before it happened.

Truth be told, I am not sure I even *want* to be allowed into my husband's innermost thoughts any longer, and so I simply rested my head against his shoulder, turned my attention back to the penguin documentary, and felt relieved when, after a few minutes, we were both laughing about how we'd gladly swap our third experience of IVF for a few months spent bracing ourselves against an Antarctic blizzard while we sat on our egg, tried not to die of exposure and waited for our little chick to hatch.

If only IVF could be so wonderfully undemanding.

12.30am

I can't sleep.

In eleven days' time I'm going to take a pregnancy test, and there is only one result that I can bring myself to contemplate.

I've already purchased my supply of pregnancy tests for the momentous occasion, and tonight I've stashed them beneath the chest of drawers that sits behind the computer in our spare bedroom (i.e. a very awkward place for me to access).

I know from past experience that I can't keep them in the bathroom cabinet and watch them winking at me suggestively every time I nip to the loo.

Over the last few years I've developed what can only be described as a deep-seated phobia of the home pregnancy test kit. Just watching the seemingly relentless adverts for the newest, most sophisticated brands that can tell you exactly how pregnant you are, presumably as well as your baby's gender, star sign and future IQ, is enough to leave me feeling physically sick.

For one insane second when I watch these adverts, my heart skips a beat, as it occurs to me that maybe, just maybe, I've stumbled across something that might help us. As though maybe I've been pregnant every time I've tested in the past, but it's just that those poxy, rubbish, substandard tests have failed me, and maybe even duped my body into reabsorbing the foetus it was actually carrying all along. But these state-of-the-art digital tests, they might work for me, like the regular ones work for everyone else. These ones might, backed by all the latest scientific technology, just give me the answer I've been waiting for at last.

Unfortunately for me, I've many times tried these bloody digital tests, and it's for them that I now reserve my most venomous pregnancy-test-induced hatred. It's the way they pretend to make it so easy for you by screaming 'NOT PREGNANT' right in your face. In my opinion, the message that pops up across the display window might as well read: 'STILL INFERTILE', 'WHAT, YOU THOUGHT YOU WERE PREGNANT? SERIOUSLY? HA HA HA HA HA!' Or perhaps the news should simply be delivered via a symbol that flashes up across the screen to give you the virtual finger.

No, I'm much more old school in my approach these days; I'd far rather grant myself the moments of uncertainty while I wait to interpret the blue or pink lines of the archetypal test stick, tilt it this way and that under the harshest of lights, and then finally break it apart like a madwoman to prove its obvious defectiveness.

Oh, crap; just *thinking* about the prospect of taking a pregnancy test leaves me feeling like I'll never sleep again. I always knew this would be the problem with treatment number three. It's why I was so desperate for treatment number two to work; I didn't ever want to find myself staring down the barrel of this gun.

Before our first IVF treatment two years ago, DH and I agreed that we would do three rounds of this invasive treatment and then no more. If we still didn't have a baby after that, we would walk away and move on with our lives.

Well, it turns out it's a lot easier to impose that kind of 'three strikes and we're out' rule upon yourself while you're still convinced that strikes one or two will meet with success.

Now that we're in the midst of the dreaded third round, I've realised that we're not just doing this to have a family; we're doing it to bring this chapter of our lives to a close.

Do we believe it's going to be third time lucky?

DH says he does, but then he's been one hundred and ten per cent positive about every treatment we've ever had, and his track record of accurately guessing the outcome hasn't been exactly shit-hot to date.

As for me, I'm starting to feel a depressing affinity with the bankrupt couple standing on the curb side, the lottery ticket that they bought with their very last pennies turning limp inside their sweating palms, justifying their final purchase by mumbling, 'Well, someone's gotta win, haven't they?'

But then, was there ever any way to avoid the two weeks that lie ahead of us?

Win or lose, I had to find out whether one more round of this awful treatment was all it was going to take. And, win or lose, ready or not, finding out is what we're now going to do.

Day Four – Friday 3rd February

Nobody Say the C Word!

Symptoms: Shooting pains up the backside (due to trapped wind), bloating, a shivery feeling as though my bowels are going to explode every time I allow thoughts of tomorrow to enter my head, and a strong desire to leave the country.

Hours until testing: 264
Waking hours until testing: 176
Predicted odds on this working: 3/10

7.30am

So, the good news is that today I get to really spice things up for myself!

For the last three days I've been inserting pessaries morning and night to boost my progesterone levels and ensure that my body is in the optimal state to receive our returning embryos – and now I get to turn those pessaries into suppositories, to make absolutely certain there will be no residue clogging the runway for tomorrow's transfer.

The downside to using the 'baby tunnel', I've found, is the sheer mess you're left with as the waxy coating of the pessary works its way out into your underwear over the course of the day. The downside to using the 'chocolate factory' is the fact that the medication then makes you even more constipated and bloated than you were when you were using the baby tunnel.

I've been told by the nurses that I'm welcome to plump for either portal from here on in, so I'm thinking maybe I'll alternate for the remaining ten days to keep things fresh and exciting.

In more pressing matters, I'm not sure I want to be around for tomorrow morning's call from Steve, when he'll tell us whether any of our five embryos have survived and are available for transfer. I've started to fantasise about packing a suitcase, switching off my phone and heading off to the nearest airport to fly anywhere in the world that isn't here.

But I know I have to somehow power through this last leg of the journey. If some of our embryos have survived, then it's my duty to cheer them on for the next ten days – no matter what Steve might tell me about them tomorrow.

He can tell me they are the poorest quality embryos he's ever seen in his life and I know I must not shed a tear. Mothers believe in their children until the bitter end; they just *know* they'll come good even in spite of the mountainous evidence to the contrary.

Well, it isn't easy being a mother to these hypothetical, ethereal babies, but it is a role I must fulfil.

9.45am

I'm concerned about how intensely cold it is outside. The latest weather update confirms it's just 2°C out there, and the air contains an Arctic chill that reminds me of a mini-break we took in Iceland in 2007. Is it possible to get pregnant in these freezing temperatures, I wonder. I don't know why, but I've always imagined I might be more fertile in warmer climes, as opposed to when I'm pacing around feeling chilled to the bone with my shoulders hunched up around my ears.

Of course, all the 'relaxation and fertility-inducing' holidays we've taken over the last few years, to places such as Greece, Spain and Thailand, reveal this not to be the case, but it doesn't stop me from feeling super infertile in these perishing conditions.

On the to-do list that I'd compiled for this two-week wait, I'd planned to take a walk every day, so as to keep myself moving, keep my blood pumping, and keep my thoughts from knotting together to form a brain-imploding mass.

Now I can't help worrying that our little embryos will be petrified within me the minute I set foot outside.

11.35pm

As I was wandering through the town centre earlier, wrapped up in scarf, hat and gloves, I was reminded of all the national celebrations that are fast approaching. In particular, Valentine's Day, which is the day of our official test and therefore a day that will forever be remembered as either the greatest or worst Valentine's Day of all time.

If this Valentine's Day were to have a crap-off contest with all the crap Valentines that have preceded it, this one could easily take first place – even *including* the one in 1992, where I spent two days beforehand gluing red and pink glitter onto a hand-designed card for a boy called Daniel Drake, who was a whole two years above me at school and evidently didn't realise I existed.

And then seven days after Valentine's Day comes Shrove Tuesday; much better than Valentine's Day in my opinion since the celebration doesn't prohibit whole chunks of the population from taking part, and who doesn't enjoy a good pancake?

But how can *I* enjoy a good pancake if we're just emerging from our third and supposedly final failed IVF treatment? By the time we reach Pancake Day, I'll either be out on the streets of London, joyfully flipping free pancakes for passing strangers, or lying in my pyjamas, flipping a coin to determine whether the dog we never wanted will be a Jack Russell or a greyhound (I'm thinking probably a greyhound at the moment because, let's face it, we may need this dog to earn its keep).

Then after Pancake Day looms Mother's Day, Easter and my birthday, followed by Father's Day, DH's birthday and finally Christmas. It's started to feel as though the year is constructed in this way purely to spite us, just to guarantee that each and every seemingly innocuous season can offer its own unique brand of torture, and whisper a snide aside to us, whilst everyone else is busy celebrating, that *yes*, another twelve months have slipped us by, and *no*, this will not be the year when we finally get to join in.

Already I can feel the weight of next Christmas bearing down on me and we're not even halfway through the second month of the year.

Of course, if we're thinking positively about the future (not something I'm often inclined to do these days), then this Christmas could be the most jubilant festive period we've ever experienced. It could see us living out scenes worthy of any Christmas card, scenes that I can only envision in my wildest daydreams right now. It could see us raising a toast around a happy family table in honour of our new arrival, and DH standing, cradling our newborn as we both stare wistfully out of the window at falling snowflakes.

Alternatively, if our worst fears are soon realised, it could see me swigging back a bottle of sherry at 7.00am in order to simply get through the day and then by lunchtime joining my grandmother's cat under the Christmas tree to nibble at some plastic pine needles and see which one of us can be first to chomp through a fairy light when the electricity is turned on.

I'm not sure I have it in me to survive another Christmas without a baby, without even a bump. And I certainly can't withstand another Christmas as gruesome as last year's – a Christmas I spent sitting in the dentist's chair having a wisdom tooth slowly and agonisingly wrenched out.

It had started to niggle a few days earlier and I was becoming convinced that if I didn't sort it out before this IVF treatment got going, there was a slim possibility I might end up needing to have it removed while I was pregnant.

I then spent Christmas Day, Boxing Day and the following two weeks drinking liquidised 'festive' root vegetables through a straw, whilst looking like a hamster that had pouched a ping-pong ball. As I sat in bed listening to the Queen's speech and nursing my roast-dinner-and-aspirin-flavoured smoothie, I took a moment to ponder which bodily part I might volunteer to have ripped out next, just on the off-chance it might otherwise choose an inopportune nine-month timeframe in which to malfunction: my tonsils, maybe? Both of my big toenails? My appendix?

To say I have come to hate the celebration we know as Christmas would truly be an understatement, and I especially hate the way it rams it home to me just how much precious time has already been lost. All those tiny little babies, conceived and born in the time we've been trying, now walking and talking and peering into cots containing their little brothers and sisters.

Our friends' and family members' years are racing past in a blur of sleepless nights, bottle feeds and bedtime stories. So much happens in the space of a year, and everywhere we look other people's lives are changing so fast.

At times like this I feel overwhelmed by the urgent need to join them, to take control, to do whatever it takes to get pregnant and have our longed-for baby before another month or year can slip through our fingers. But the frustrating truth is that we're already doing all we can and going as fast as we can – and it still doesn't bring us any closer.

If the ghost of Christmas future asked me to look into a crystal ball today, I know I'd have my hands up over my eyes and would only be able to peep out from between the cracks in my fingers, because I'm just scared to death of what, or rather *who*, won't be sitting round the family table for all those end-of-year celebrations that are to come.

3.00pm

As scheduled several weeks ago, I met my friend Sally for lunch this afternoon in a small café close to London's South Bank. She knows we're gearing up for another round of IVF at some point in the near future, but she doesn't know we're actually halfway through it right now; the details of this experience, as I've already learned, are mostly better left unshared.

By the time Sally arrived, I had already ordered two peppermint teas and a giant slice of strawberry cheesecake for us to carve up over the next couple of hours. It is a ten-year-long tradition of ours that for each of our rendezvous we will seek out some previously undiscovered cake shop and order the most calorific offering on the menu.

'You still eating this stuff, then?' Sally laughed as she gave me a big hug and unwound her stripy winter scarf. 'I thought you'd be on some kind of organic, lentil-and-spinach-only diet by now.'

I was sure I caught a hint of recrimination in her voice, and it reminded me of how I've grown to loathe other people's scrutiny of each tiny corner of my life. In particular, I've noticed some of my single friends, like Sally, taking an unhealthy interest in the dietary and lifestyle choices I've made throughout my life.

Sometimes I get the impression that they're trying to build a profile of the infertile woman, to make a mental note of where they think I screwed up, and how they might prevent themselves from realising the same fate.

It's a fact that no woman of childbearing age who plans on having a family wants to find any common ground with me anymore.

'Don't worry, I can get really bad stomach cramps when it's that time of the month,' I might say, or, 'It's okay, I always feel that way before a period, too. I think it's normal.'

Their horrified, wordless gapes convey it all. It most definitely is not all right, or normal, because I am most definitely neither of those things.

I don't blame them for reacting this way, to be honest. Sharing any kind of reproductive trait with me must be like describing your recent aches and pains to someone and then having them turn around and inform you that they experienced the *very* same sensations right before being rushed off to A&E with their first stroke.

'I have news,' Sally told me almost as soon as she sat down, reaching across the table and grasping my hands in hers.

'Oh holy fucking crap, please don't you fucking dare tell me you're pregnant!' I wanted to scream in her face, before reassuring myself that the chances of that, given that Sally was single last time I saw her six weeks ago, had to be vanishingly small.

I still held my breath and pressed my legs hard against the underside of the table while I waited for her to continue.

'I've met someone,' she told me, excitedly. 'His name's Tom, he doesn't appear to be a psychopath or a knobhead, and I don't know…I kind of think this might go somewhere.'

Sally carried on talking, telling me all about Tom: how they'd met three weeks ago in a bar opposite her work, how he was thirty-seven, came out of a ten-year relationship twelve months ago and was really eager to meet the right woman, settle down and have a couple of kids.

Oh *shit*, I found myself thinking, desperately. I bet he's got super sperm, too; I bet he's got the kind of sperm count that could repopulate Russia. *And* the bastard wants to unleash it. Oh fuck, they're going to do it, aren't they? They're going to have one of those whirlwind romances people have where they go from single and renting a studio flat one minute, to getting married, moving into a five-bedroomed detached house and getting pregnant with twins the next. Sally herself is a twin. Oh my god, Sally is going to grab hold of Tom by his super, spunk-packed bollocks and get herself knocked up with twins, isn't she? And by the time her twins are enrolled in nursery, I'll still be ~~childless~~ childfree and barren and probably living in a squat because we'll have surrendered our flat in pursuit of more failed fertility treatments. Oh Jesus, fucking… SHIT.

I tried to halt that particular train of thought before I found myself a hyperventilating wreck on the floor. And then I forced myself to focus on how nice it was to see my friend (yes, my *friend*) so sparkly-eyed and happy and alive.

And I tried to hope that it *did* work out for Sally and Tom. I wanted to hope that they did just fall madly in love, settle down and have a beautiful family: one girl (with Sally's pretty elfin face, bobbed red hair and undeniable brains) and one boy (with Tom's rugged good looks and life-affirming heroism and charm – I was making a few assumptions here, but he was bound to be almost superhuman, wasn't he?). Sally deserved some happiness after all, and she certainly deserved better than a rotten, miserable friend who couldn't even be remotely excited for her that she'd been out on a few successful dates.

I hate myself sometimes, I honestly do.

Later in the afternoon, after I'd said goodbye to Sally and taken myself for a long walk beside the Thames, the glacial February wind in my hair, I vowed to refrain from tutting at all the tired-out career women with 'baby on board' badges proudly stuck to their coats, and from scowling at the unborn babies they carried within their fully functioning wombs. But it was no use. I could not pretend to feel goodwill towards the pregnant members of womankind, and my bitterness consumed me, turned me away from the rest of the world and in on myself, as it inevitably always does.

Stepping through the front door of our flat, I realised I had become so preoccupied by my own mental turmoil that I couldn't remember a single detail about the journey I had just taken; the streets could have been paved with injured animals, abandoned children and homeless pensioners, and I would have stormed right past them all, mumbling angrily under my breath about how cruel and unjust this shitty world can be.

This is not what was supposed to happen to me, I can't help but think every day; this is SO not the woman that I ever thought I would become.

7.45pm

DH arrived home an hour ago after what sounds like a diabolical day at work; one of those days that is crammed to capacity with rude requests, unrealistic expectations and ungrateful arseholes with far more money than manners. And now, to top it off, I have just attempted to poison him with an undercooked chicken.

I can't help but worry that other women in my situation (childless childfree housewives with nothing to occupy their time, that is) would be doing a much better job. Surely I should be some sort of domestic goddess by now, dancing round this flat with a feather duster each morning, and then rustling up a Michelin star three-course banquet each night. Oh, how I preferred it when things were equal and balanced, when DH and I both arrived home at night, shattered from a hard day's work, and took it in turns to simply slip a ready meal into the oven.

DH didn't complain, of course, just headed off into the kitchen to see if he could salvage his half-raw bird, but I know he must be wondering if there is any task in the world that wouldn't prove too much for me these days. I can't have his babies, I can't go out to work, if tonight's anything to go by I sure as hell can't cook, and of course sex if off the menu pretty much all the time. Just as well I'm married, I suppose, because my personal ad would not be attracting much attention if I had to get back on the dating scene right now.

10.30pm

Oh, for fuck's sake.

My friend Jane has just emailed me an invite to her twins' second birthday party next Saturday. She says it will be a great opportunity for a catch-up (once all the other kids have gone home), and since her mother's there to look after the twins and their older brother, she'll be hitting the wine at five o'clock and it'll be just like old times.

Well, not for me it won't, Jane! It won't be like the old times or the new times; it'll just be an extension of the crap times in which I now reside.

This godforsaken party will also inevitably be filled with familiar old faces and vague acquaintances – people who have the power to steamroller, quite obliviously, across the most sensitive landscape of my life.

A truthful question-and-answer session with this endless stream of tosspots, if I imagine it in my head, would have to go something like this:

Them: Oh hi there, how are you?

Me: Oh, you know, depressed, poor, unemployed, infertile, can't complain really.

Them: You still working at that marketing company in the City?

Me: No, I voluntarily left last year. And yes, I really did do that with no other work to go on to, no savings in my bank account, and no clue about what to do next.

Them: How's the other half? Still working as a freelance IT consultant, is he?

Me: Well, technically yes, although he's only had one job in the last five months since he turned down a really good project in order to spend the day wanking into a small plastic cup.

Them: Oh, right. How long have you guys been married now?

Me: Five years now. Yes, you heard that right: five *years*.

Them: Any kids?

Me: No, but we're thinking of getting a greyhound because, you know, we live in a tiny London flat without even a balcony and, more importantly, we both really hate dogs.

Them: So, you checking out anywhere interesting on your travels this year?

Me: Well, I guess that depends on how interesting you find the hospital theatres of fertility clinics in our country's capital…

From now on, to avoid this kind of awkwardness, and in recognition of the fact that I'm such an unconventional, confusing enigma to people who attempt small talk with me, I've decided to make social interactions less painful for everyone concerned and simply start lying.

Until I have a baby or reach menopause, I will forever now be twenty-nine, married almost a year and working hard in my last job. I don't care how implausible it starts to sound, because the one benefit of speaking to vague acquaintances is that it takes an extraordinarily rude one to question the authenticity of your answers.

But I can't cope with any of this bullshit right now. I can't risk 'innocent' conversations with strangers and I can't listen to Jane advising me that if I were to spend more time with other pregnant women and mothers then I would instantaneously become pregnant myself, presumably through some form of osmosis. I can't smile at her pleasantly as she tells me, one twin balanced on either hip, that she understands *exactly* how I feel because it took her an angst-ridden five months to conceive her firstborn. And I most definitely can't promise I won't punch her out cold if she instructs me to go travelling, set up my own business or adopt a Romanian orphan, on the grounds that pregnancy is only ever going to come about now when I'm least expecting it to happen.

I mean, if that were true then I should really undergo a hysterectomy, join a nunnery or leave DH and become a lesbian. Because if I were to get pregnant in *those* circumstances, it really would qualify as an incredible bloody surprise, wouldn't it?

Naturally, there is a big, no *huge*, part of me that *wants* to go and spend some quality time with my friends. But I know by now what happens at the end of these sorts of get-togethers: the parents go away feeling gratified that they've found the time to catch up and squeeze in some much missed 'adult time' with their ~~childless~~ childfree friends. And I go away and contemplate sticking my head in the oven.

'So don't go, then,' DH said, matter-of-factly, when I confessed my latest dilemma to him.

But the offer isn't that easy to decline, I tried to explain. I don't want to be the bitter old recluse who thinks that she's the only person in the world with problems. I don't want to be the woman who just yawns and snaps, 'Yeah, well, at least you've got kids!' if at any point in the future Jane confides in me that her mother-in-law's moving in with her and her husband appears to be having an affair with his squash partner, Mark.

'Right. So, don't be that person, then,' DH said, momentarily glancing up from his laptop. 'Go to the party.'

I shook my head and sighed. 'Haven't you been listening to a SINGLE WORD I've said to you?' I barked at him.

'Look, you're just worried about tomorrow,' DH told me, a somewhat patronising tone entering his voice.

'Of course I am,' I yelled over my shoulder as I headed to the kitchen to grab a third helping of Brazil nuts. 'So should you be! I don't know why the hell you're so relaxed.'

'Third time lucky,' he called after me. 'It'll all be fine.'

Of course. The immortal words uttered by men all over the world every single day: 'It'll all be fine!'

Well, why didn't I think of that?

My current fertility counsellor (the one who came free as part of the £6,500 IVF package with our latest clinic) suggested that DH has been forced to adopt the 'glass half full' outlook on our situation, purely because it just wouldn't be workable for both halves of a partnership to be as negative as I am!

Where there is night, there must also be day, she explained, and in these testing sink-or-swim predicaments, it is normal for somebody to cast themselves as the rock, the pillar of strength, the cheerleader.

I know deep down that she is right. And I also feel curious to know how DH *really* feels right now, what he truly believes or fears will happen.

But, interestingly, I guess I've never felt curious enough to actually ask the question. Maybe I need his boundless optimism more than I'd care to admit, and maybe the honest truth is that there are some home truths and honest answers that I may never be ready to hear.

And so, for tonight, I will try to stop talking, stop worrying and stop thinking.

I will force down some more fertility-boosting brazil nuts with a glass of fertility-boosting full-fat milk, and then I will hold DH close, I will breathe him in, and I will try to let his confidence seep beneath my skin.

I will try to believe him when he tells me that the planets are aligning, the tides are a-turning, and that better things are surely now heading our way.

Day Five – Saturday 4th February

Let It Snow

Symptoms: A healthy smattering of embarrassment given the thousand-watt bulb that's about to illuminate my lady garden in a room full of strangers. But the good thing about the embryo transfer, I've discovered, is that I tend to be so distracted by the thought of the embryos themselves that it's easy to ignore the undignified position in which I've once again found myself.

Hours until testing: 240

Waking hours until testing: 160

Predicted odds of this working: 9.9/10

7.45am

Well, what a difference a day makes.

I'm sat here with a cup of lemon and ginger tea, trying to savour the last few hours of being on my own before I become a vessel for our precious cargo for what I hope is the next nine months.

In a few hours' time I'll be a little bit pregnant, at least halfway towards a positive pregnancy test, and a good few steps closer to screaming down a labour ward at some point towards the end of this year.

Steve, our wonderful, extraordinary, miracle-performing embryologist, has already called to tell us that two of our embryos are still going strong, which means today's scheduled transfer is definitely going ahead.

So, this is it. We've been granted another chance, another roll of the dice; one last opportunity to win favour with Lady Luck.

Just two more hours and we get to bring our embryos (our *babies*) home.

2.20pm

We made it back to the house just minutes before the first proper snow of this winter started to fall.

There's something a little romantic about being snowed in with our new little embryos hopefully snuggled up in the warm – but then everything is verging on downright magical just now. If I were to open a speeding fine in the post, drop my keys down a drain or retrieve my favourite cream jumper from a wash containing a rogue red sock, I'd just smile and think about how charmingly mischievous the world can be.

I wish I could bottle this feeling and slow-release it over the next nine days.

If someone had told me at the start of this treatment that I'd have felt as positively about its potential outcome as I do at this moment, I'd never have believed it possible. I felt certain I'd be going through the motions, resigned to failure from the very beginning. And yet, as I was changing into my rather fetching hospital gown, hairnet and slippers this morning and the nurse asked me whether I was feeling excited, my bitter alter-ego didn't, as I'd have expected, glare at her and ask her how excited *she'd* be feeling right now if she were in my shoes. Instead I found myself smiling at her and nodding, a sense of genuine elation fluttering in my stomach.

The capacity for human hope really is astounding.

Now that we're safely within the confines of the house, I can finally breathe a sigh of relief that we've made it back from the hospital without being seen.

Since we have decided to keep this treatment entirely under wraps, I've been constantly paranoid about bumping into someone we know, particularly on a day like today when it would be impossible to hide the fact that something completely out of the ordinary is going on.

There's a certain walk reserved for a very limited range of situations in life. It's the walk I'll be walking for the rest of today and it reveals to everyone around me one of several possibilities:

I'm a drug mule, rectally smuggling huge quantities of cocaine into the country.

I've just very suddenly and catastrophically soiled my underwear.

I'm going through IVF and have just had my eggs collected or...

I'm going through IVF and have just had my embryos transferred.

In each of these scenarios (I'm imagining, of course, as I've only actually experienced three of them), a woman is seen taking miniature, shuffling steps forwards, her back rigid, her buttocks clenched, a look of wild panic and yet intense concentration betraying the frantic internal dialogue that's taking place inside her head.

The final two IVF-related walks are actually very similar; it's just that during the first one a woman is physically unable to walk, and during the second she's simply too scared of gravity to get to her feet.

It makes no sense whatsoever, but I feel that our embryos are so delicately balanced within my body that they might drop out at any second. I feel that if I were to hop, skip, slip over, cough, sneeze, blow my nose or even fart in an over-zealous fashion, they would be expelled from my vagina instantaneously.

Logically, I know this can't happen, and I also know that our transfer was 'textbook perfect' – well, as perfect as an embryo transfer could ever be, that is.

I mean, naturally, as Dr Rangan greeted us this afternoon, I did have to try *very* hard to erase the image of our last encounter from my mind: Dr Rangan's head hovering somewhere between my inner thighs, his nose practically skimming my labia as he carefully extracted my eggs via a tiny, needle-like instrument.

To give our consultant his due, he does a sterling job of pretending all that nose-to-labia stuff never actually happened. Well, a much better job than I'd do if the last time we'd met I'd been standing over him in a harshly lit room, fishing stuff out of the end of his wiener.

But every woman knows that the embarrassment factor is not what really matters during the transfer. The major concern for the IVF patient is whether or not the embryos are actually *in* her by the end of the procedure. Obviously, the embryologist always checks the catheter under a microscope both before and after the transfer, to make sure they haven't been either released or retained at the wrong moment – but I still can't help worrying that they somehow ended up on the floor.

I hadn't realised before we began fertility treatment that embryos were so terrifyingly small. But now I know that each one is roughly the size of a speck of dust, it's easy to imagine how accidents could happen.

We even had to sign a form before the transfer took place, accepting that human error *might* occur and that – very, very rarely – an embryo might become, well, 'lost' during a transfer.

I guess all it would take is a sudden sneeze, a little wobble, a bit of a hangover maybe and whoopsie! Just like that, the precious embryo – quite possibly the *one* precious embryo that had been created after months of preparation, weeks of injections and one very painful extraction – could be relegated to the underside of an embryologist's shoe.

'Oops-a-daisy!' Dr Rangan might exclaim under his breath. 'Butter fingers strike again.'

Or maybe nobody would actually have the guts to tell us in that situation.

'Oh yes, that's gone in just fine,' they'd probably grin, reassuring themselves that I'm a patient who never gets pregnant anyway so it most likely won't make a scrap of difference.

But this isn't a very comforting train of thought to pursue, so I'm just going to have to convince myself that Dr Rangan was telling the truth when he assured us that this embryo transfer was 'absolutely fine'.

My only wish, in retrospect, is that it had occurred to him to install some kind of internal camera at the same time, so that I could now sit here at home, hook up a monitor to our 46-inch plasma screen, and spend the next nine days studying the inner developments taking place.

Imagine it: it would be like watching a week-long World Cup final, second by agonising nail-biting second. We could invite round all our friends and family to perch on the edge of the sofa and cheer on our embryos if it looked as though they were going to win, or leap to their feet, clasp the sides of their heads, scream at the TV screen and smash up the living room if it looked as though they were heading for defeat.

Or, better still, Dr Rangan could have gone one step further when he set up the internal camera and given me a remote control to accompany the monitor. Then I could put all those years of playing *Street Fighter* as a student to good use, and use my super-strong nimble thumbs to bust those embryos into my uterus, no matter how many evil antibodies or other enemies I needed to karate chop into oblivion before they were safe.

Before the transfer went ahead, we had the usual lively discussion about how many embryos we should put back this time. Just like last time and the time before, the team was adamant that, as it was a blastocyst transfer, it must be only the one, because the chances of conceiving twins was otherwise too great.

It's a perplexing fact in IVF that while we're worrying ourselves sick about not becoming pregnant at all, the consultants at our clinics are worried about us going too far, overshooting the mark and ending up with a double whammy or even a hat-trick.

But why would any consultant waste even an ounce of mental energy on worrying about something like that happening to us?

'You do realise how bad at this I am, don't you?' I checked with them before we went ahead.

I mean, I think my track record speaks for itself. And, to be truthful, in my most pessimistic moments I reckon we could probably transfer nine hundred and ninety-nine embryos to my womb and still come out the other end with a negative pregnancy test in our hands.

It always seems so cruel that these professionals ask us to seriously contemplate the dangers of a multiple pregnancy when my body has been so immune and averse to any sort of pregnancy up until now.

Also, I have to admit, in spite of the risks that we're aware of, we'd be nothing short of ecstatic to find ourselves pregnant with twins. I mean, obviously we are saying that from a position of deep naivety, since we have no idea what carrying, giving birth to and bringing up twins would actually entail.

The trouble is, no matter how many times you're told otherwise, when you've lived with the very real fear that you may never have a baby at all, it's hard to see the possibility of suddenly acquiring two of them as anything other than a pretty fantastic outcome.

In the end, DH and I managed to persuade Steve and Dr

Rangan, just as we persuaded the staff at our previous clinics, that in this instance replacing two embryos was a reasonable 'risk' to take.

And now, with our two embryos on board, I'm determined to believe it's all going to work out this time.

We were unlucky on the last two cycles, so the chances are we should be lucky this time, right? I mean, if this is all just a random game of chance, then what are the odds of flipping three tails in a row?

One in eight, I've just learned, following a quick, maths-based Internet search.

One in eight is pretty good odds. And I realise that this is not at all how it works with IVF, but I'm just going to tell myself that there's a seven in eight chance that we are almost certainly going to flip a head this time.

4.45pm

Okay, so I feel ludicrous admitting this, even to myself, but I have just dug out a little lucky mascot from its secret hiding place in my bedside drawer, and I've prayed that it might bring me some good fortune over the next nine days. The mascot in question is a small pink fertility crystal pendant, sent to me three months ago by my good friend and mother of three, Jane.

I remember she had prefaced its arrival by saying that she knew I would be cynical, and I'm pretty sure that my response at the time didn't disappoint. In fact, I near enough jumped down her throat, telling her that since our fertility problems lay beyond the restorative powers of the most advanced medical treatments, I feared we would be something of a tall order for the likes of a small pink crystal. A tall order, like having the lower half of your leg bitten off by a shark and hoping that, by placing a circle of healing crystals around the bleeding stump, it might just grow back again.

Jane told me that it had only been a thought; she wouldn't send it after all.

But then a couple of months went by and I experienced something that I had never experienced before: a late period! The hope and excitement that surfaced within, followed by the despair of yet another negative pregnancy test and the eventual arrival of the absent period, crushed me almost as systematically as our failed IVF treatments.

That was last November and just one month before this final IVF cycle was set to begin. DH was bracing himself for the blow of another birthday, we were galloping towards another Christmas, and then – the final straw – another pregnancy in the family was announced. That was it. I cracked.

'Send me the healing fertility crystal!' I begged Jane via a 3.00am text one Saturday morning.

She had popped it through my letterbox the very next day, with a kind note saying she hoped it would bring me good luck. It was a much kinder note than the one I deserved, which would have said something along the lines of hoping that instead of a *leg*, my grouchy old *head* had been bitten off by a shark and that the fertility crystal might help me to grow a newer, more pleasant one in its place.

Of course, I still can't fully believe that I begged my friend for a healing fertility crystal, or that I'm sitting here wearing it now. And I wish I could go back to a time when I could confidently dismiss this sort of thing as utter codswallop. But those days are long gone now.

So many times I've unearthed a story about some woman who's tried one of these things and become pregnant after seventeen years of trying, and I can't quite find the resolve within myself not to wonder, 'What if?'

And it's this niggling 'what if' that has seen me resort to a whole host of things over the years: acupuncture, reflexology, positive visualisation, every vitamin and supplement under the sun, herbal tinctures, fertility-boosting shakes, the consumption of brazil nuts and kiwi fruit and pineapple cores (it's a wonder there isn't a pineapple crown sprouting from the top of my head by now), the guzzling of full-fat milk, the wearing of orange knickers, and so the list goes on…

But does eating, drinking and doing all this stuff actually contribute to getting pregnant? Almost certainly not, but who cares? At this stage in the game I'm not ashamed to admit I no longer have much interest in pinpointing exactly what has worked for us, and why. It's more a case of slinging as much mud or, in this instance, as many crystals, milky drinks and pineapple cores at my uterine wall as possible, and just hoping that the magical combination of it all somehow makes an embryo stick.

9.47pm

Well, I'm just about ready to turn in. I've done nothing for the last nine hours but lie on the sofa, but somehow it's still felt like the most exhausting of days.

And unlike the days following my egg retrieval, when I sat in bed scoffing a packet of Jaffa cakes, my body is now back to being an organic temple. Or a Fabergé egg that might shatter at the slightest nudge.

But, in spite of the immense responsibility, it feels wonderful to be a fragile Fabergé egg, to be the sacred carrier of two potential little babies once more.

And, in the spirit of glowing optimism, DH and I have tonight decided to temporarily name our two potential little babies Kenneth and Donaghy, after our favourite characters in the US comedy series *30 Rock*. We've agreed that we'll come up with something more suitable before their births (particularly if they turn out to be girls), but for now we figure that if any of our embryos are ever going to make it, then these two upbeat little entities will be the ones to blaze the trail.

Already, I've found myself rubbing my belly protectively and talking to Kenneth and Donaghy, instructing them in what they'll need to do over the next few days, just in case they feel confused and unsure about what comes next.

And, in turn, DH has tried to reassure *me* that all *I* need to do is to stay calm for the next two hundred and forty-eight hours and to prevent my mind from being overtaken by fears and superstitions, or worries about what I believe might be good or bad omens.

'If you catch sight of two single magpies, but in a very short space of time, do you think that counts as one helping of joy or just a double helping of sorrow?' I had asked him during our drive home from the clinic this afternoon.

He had rolled his eyes in response; he knows me too well to be surprised by this kind of question now. He knows that I'll be obsessed with avoiding any lone black-and-white birds over the next nine days, and that I'll be casually stalking all the black cats in the neighbourhood, just in the hope that one might turn around and deign to cross my path.

'Look, important things are happening in there,' he told me earlier this evening, nodding in the direction of my womb. 'And nothing that takes place in the world out here can stop those things from happening now.'

I suppose I know deep down that he is right. I mean, so what if I really were to be stalked by a lone magpie, who swooped down, perched atop my shoulder and insisted on accompanying me every-where I went? Or if we wake tomorrow morning to find an angry swarm of locusts encircling our flat? Or if the neighbourhood black cat *does* deign to cross my path, but chooses to do so under the cover of nightfall and whilst I'm performing my usual seventeen-point manoeuvre to get out of our parking space, leaving it seventeen times flattened and welded to the tarmac like a scorched, furry pancake?

Because even if one of these things really *were* to happen, in fact even if *all* of these things were to happen, one after the other in a relentless stream of bad omens over the next nine days, it still doesn't change anything, does it? It still couldn't change the fact that Kenneth and Donaghy, our two little somethings, the size of specks of dust, have been selected as life forces with which to be reckoned.

After all, a lot of the hard work has already been done. All Kenneth and Donaghy have to do now is hatch out of their shells, burrow deep inside my uterus and then grow, grow and grow into something with two arms, two legs, a heart and a brain and a unique collaboration of abilities, anxieties and character quirks.

It seems a lot to ask of a tiny cluster of cells. But then every human alive must have looked like Kenneth and Donaghy once upon a time, and we all managed to get here somehow.

So, all I can do now, my little warriors, is wish you the very best of luck. And to reassure myself that, if your father managed to accomplish this mission, then it can't have required too much in the way of organisational prowess, so there should be no reason why you can't accomplish it, too.

Oh, and please don't be deterred by all that stuff you might have picked up on today about crystals and black cats and magpies, will you?

I promise you there's still a chance your mother may not always sound like the corduroy-wearing, chanting, hippy fruitcake you might mistake her for this evening.

Day Six — Sunday 5th February

A Virtual Reality

Symptoms: The odd twinge in my right ovary, sore boobs (which I know are a direct result of the pessaries and suppositories I'm using morning and night) and an inability to focus on anything for longer than five seconds.

Hours until testing: 216
Waking hours until testing: 144
Predicted odds of this working: 5/10

6.30am

Well, it's not even light outside and already this day is off to a most disastrous start.

I stumbled through to the bathroom at the ungodly hour of 6.00am, went for a wee, walked over to wash my hands in the sink and caught a glimpse of my healing fertility crystal plummeting from my chest towards the sink and then vanishing down the plughole.

Oh. Jesus. Christ.

I know DH would argue otherwise, but could there ever be a more definitive portent of doom?

Part of me wants to call Dr Rangan's secretary right now and leave a message explaining that this cycle is all over, because there's clearly no sense in carrying any hope for the final outcome now.

7.50am

Okay, so it would appear that the world-ending cataclysm has been averted. Having spent ten minutes unscrewing the metal plug and frantically fishing through the black gooey crud inside the plughole, I've succeeded in rescuing the rose quartz pendant, which, following a good scrub, is safely fastened on its silver chain and back around my neck.

'Phew,' I said loudly, plonking myself down heavily on the end of the bed.

'Yeah, thank fuck for that,' DH muttered into his pillow in a not entirely supportive tone.

I realise that he must seem like the sane, rational half of our partnership right now, but I wish he'd be a bit more sympathetic to my neurotic, unhinged brain sometimes.

9.30am

We were reawakened at 8.30am by the final call from Steve, telling us that, having battled through the seven inches of snow that have settled overnight to check on our remaining embryos, none of the stragglers, classified yesterday as 'early blastocysts', has developed any further. Regretfully, he tells us, this means there won't be any backup embryos for our personal freezer.

Oh well, it was okay, we reassured him, we knew it had been a long shot, and we also knew we should feel lucky that even two of our embryos had made it to that stage.

DH gripped my hand and we thanked Steve profusely for his valiant efforts to make a last-minute recruit to our reproductive ice box. And then I had to cut the conversation dead because I could feel an uncomfortable lump beginning to rise at the back of my throat.

This really is it, then. No backup, no contingency, no Plan B.

At best, a frozen embryo or two could have offered Kenneth and Donaghy the opportunity to have a little brother or sister at some point in the future; at the very least, it could have provided a little ray of hope, one final stop at the last-chance saloon before supposedly hanging up our IVF socks once and for all.

As we said our goodbyes, it occurred to me that DH and I will never speak to Steve again. It sounds silly, but the acknowledgement of this fact suddenly feels like a terrible wrench. And it's probably because, like all the other embryologists we've met to date, Steve has been one of the kindest people you could ever hope to encounter, the sort of person whose compassion – in the face of your utter vulnerability – almost makes you want to collapse in a heap and sob great tears of gratitude for the goodness that can still be found in mankind.

But since his role in this latest chapter of our lives is now over, I can only try to take comfort in the memory of his worried expression and his stern words of warning yesterday afternoon as he urged us to have only one embryo transferred, and told us how concerned he felt that, with one top-grade and one middle-grade blastocyst on board, he might be sending us on our merry way with a twin pregnancy in the making.

I wish more than anything that I could share his anxiety, but I'm afraid I know my uncooperative body better than he does. In fact, I can't explain exactly what has happened, but today I already feel that I'm chasing after yesterday's optimism, snatching desperately at its coattails as it disappears from the rear-view mirror.

I wish it were possible to hang on to the certainty I conjured so easily yesterday afternoon. But now that Kenneth and Donaghy are drifting, unsupervised, in the inner caverns of my body, it's so much harder to tell myself that they are definitely doing fine.

Just like children on a missing person's poster, my two little babies were last seen alive more than twenty-four hours ago, and now, until I have proof to the contrary back in front of my eyes, I can't help but fear the worst.

10.30am

Okay, I'll admit it: I decided to take a pregnancy test when I got up for the second time this morning, just to check whether or not the trigger shot (used to mature my eggs before the retrieval) was fully out of my system. Containing high levels of HCG, the hormone produced in early pregnancy, the trigger shot can reportedly linger in the body for up to fourteen days, and I was convinced there would still be at least a trace of it left in mine.

There wasn't, it turns out. If I'm honest, I was a little disappointed. As tragic as it sounds, I would have loved to see a positive pregnancy test, even though I'd have known it couldn't be for real. I'd just like to say that I've seen one, even once, if only to prove that it's possible for a pregnancy test to turn positive in my hands.

There's a bigger problem resulting from this morning's unscheduled test, though. Testing out the trigger shot now paves the way for me to be a very rebellious patient and to test much earlier than my official test date of February 14th. Had I resisted the temptation this morning, I would have known that testing early was out of the question, fearing the false positive I might have seen if the HCG trigger shot was just taking a long time to filter out of my body.

I promised myself I was not going to test early this time. Did I really need to give myself any more of a reason to violate my own good intentions?

2.20pm

For the last couple of hours I've been sat by our first-floor window, gazing down at the busy High Street beneath me and watching what has felt like an endless stream of parents ploughing through the snow with cute little snow bears strapped to their chests and slightly bigger snow bears sliding along behind them on toboggans.

These snippets of the idyllic family life are all around me, everywhere I go; even sitting here in the supposed sanctuary of my own home they can start to infiltrate from the world outside.

And I've also been picturing a parallel universe where our own little snow bears, Kenneth and Donaghy, might be taken out for some winter fun on those increasingly special and rare days of British snow.

This glimpse into a happier world – our own potential future – feels heart-warming but implausible, like a beautiful mirage that could so easily evaporate if I were to take a step too close.

6.00pm

About an hour ago I received a text message from my best friend Nat, suggesting that she could travel down from Edinburgh to stay with me for a couple of days.

It's one of the most tempting offers I can imagine right now. DH will be going back to work tomorrow, I haven't seen Nat for more than a year and, although she doesn't know what we're going through (unless my healing fertility crystal has telepathically informed her and summoned her presence, of course), it would be the most wonderful distraction to spend a couple of days laughing, catching up, being childish and generally forgetting that we ever grew up at all.

The only snag (and it's a pretty fucking big one!) is that she's also the friend who had to inform me of her second pregnancy the day after our second failed IVF cycle last year, which currently puts her at around seven and a half months pregnant.

My initial reaction is that it will surely push me over the edge to spend three days with a big pregnant belly in the middle of this two-week wait, no matter how much I might love the person to whom it is attached.

But then we *have* to see each other at some point, and the truth is, when it comes to huge pink elephants that stand boldly in the middle of the room but must still be ignored, a pregnant belly is always going to be preferable to a newborn baby.

The other inescapable reality is that I may be happier now than I'm going to be in quite some time. At least for the moment I know there's a *chance* that I might just be pregnant, too.

Perhaps what it boils down to is a practicality. Normal women get nine months to enjoy their pregnancies; some of us are given only nine days. So maybe I should simply 'buck up' and learn to be grateful for the short time I definitely have?

In some ways it makes it easier, and in some ways it makes it even more impossible, that Nat is the sort of friend who would have gladly traded her positive pregnancy test with my negative one seven and a half months ago. As it is, it wouldn't surprise me if she stepped off her coach wearing a two-man tent when we go to pick her up, just so as not to cause any upset or offence by flouting her bump.

The two of us shared some fun times in her quaint Scottish cottage during her first pregnancy four years ago. We sat round a fire until the small hours discussing everything to do with pregnancy and childbirth, flicking through a baby names book and laughing over the most outrageous monikers that she could possibly give to her firstborn.

How times change. How incredibly resentful I'm left feeling now that my infertility has robbed me not only of the joy of my own pregnancies but also of the joy of other people's. And that other people have been robbed entirely of the joy of their own pregnancies whenever they find themselves in my company.

I miss my friends sometimes. Especially the old ones, the ones I became friends with when all our futures seemed about as directionless as mine is now. But then there is so much…*life*…that prevents these old friends from socialising these days – and such a huge amount of…well, *nothing*…that prevents me from doing the same.

I've noticed that most of my friends go into a state of hibernation with their babies (just as I have without mine), emerging a couple of years later with a slightly crazed look in their eyes and talking about how *amazing* it would be to plan a night out and maybe revisit one of the old haunts that we last frequented when we were all about twenty-five.

They don't just casually suggest it either; they are possessed by the idea, determined to go there and neck ten tequila shots, get absolutely smashed and divulge endless confessions about sex after childbirth and how much they despise their husbands.

Sometimes, this kind of reintroduction to footloose living can extend to whole weekends away with the girls, if money and babysitters are in sufficiently plentiful supply.

'GOD, I really *needed* this!' everyone concludes, reaffirming for one another how imperative it is to shake off the humdrum and unglamorous reality of parental duty and to let one's hair down once in a while.

But then, inevitably, the hangover hits, and everybody realises that while it was fun to invoke their inner teenager for a night, there is now somewhere else that they would much rather be. And at some point during the last day, as we wearily wend our way home, I can see that the excitement's returning to their eyes, fuelled by the mental image of those tiny bodies that will attach to their legs like limpets as soon as their overnight bag hits the floor.

'I do hate being away from them,' they all confess on the journey back, rushing now to get home to the life they couldn't wait to escape from just a few days before.

In the world of parenthood at least, it seems absence really does make the heart grow fonder. And maybe I need to take a leaf out of their books and learn to grow fonder of some of the people and things I so often take for granted in my own ~~childless~~ childfree life.

The trouble is, no matter how I try (and, contrary to what DH believes, I *do* try) to reframe our situation and cement this ugly picture onto a prettier backdrop, I can't quite shake the feeling that I'm not yet a proper grown-up. It's as though I'm living only a fraction of a life, the sort of existence that other people can only try to relate to when they look back into the dim and distant recesses of their own histories.

Everyone knows that there are important phases of life, rites of passage through which every adult should eventually travel. Everything changes, they say. Nothing stays the same.

So how, then, can it be that my life is continually stuck on hold?

7.15pm

I just can't decide what to do about Nat.

And so, to escape the pressures and awkwardness of 'real' friendships, I've spent a full hour online, chatting to women across the globe who are currently at a similar stage in their own IVF treatments.

We are, ironically, part of a website dedicated to pregnancies, births and childcare, but we are the dark underbelly of this world, with our forums devoted to infertility treatments, recurrent miscarriages, donor eggs and sperm, and life without children.

We've each allocated ourselves an avatar from a well-known

children's story, and chosen for ourselves screen names like Goldilocks, Snow White, Ariel and Piglet.

When I first joined the forum three years ago, the names instantly brought to mind a set of characters from a Quentin Tarantino-style film. And now that I've come to know so many of the women behind the screen names, I've learned that there probably is a sufficient amount of gore and horror in some of our lives to form a suitably Tarantino-esque kind of script.

Although I've never actually met any of them face to face, Goldilocks, Snow and Ariel are the women who really 'get it', without any need for complex explanation. None of us can get pregnant for love nor money, and we should know, after all; to tackle this problem we have each by now thrown in bucket loads of both ingredients.

Right now, there are around twenty of us on the forum in the midst of our two-week waits, and we're trying our hardest to keep one another sane while, I've begun to suspect, simultaneously driving one another deeper and deeper into madness.

There has been a palpable, shared anxiety on the forum this afternoon. Piglet has had only two eggs collected, Goldilocks's DH has just lost his job, which means they probably can't afford to cycle again if this treatment doesn't work, and Snow White is feeling as though she's about to get her AF (Aunt Flo) just four days after her embryos were transferred.

Naturally, I quite enjoy immersing myself in these other women's daily updates; I guess that trying to offer them some sort of comfort and solidarity makes me feel a little less useless, gives me something (and someone) else to think about, and helps me cling to the belief that I'm perhaps not completely alone after all.

'You *do* know that they're not real?' DH continues to comment each time he catches me in the act of chatting to my Tarantino buddies online.

I don't know what he thinks they are.

I *do* understand his reluctance to lose me to the 'second life' kind of existence I've been living, but what he doesn't appreciate is that my Tarantino buddies have compensated for a great deal of shortcomings in the real world. My struggles with infertility and the level of anxiety I'm experiencing right now can, after all, only be discussed for so long within the confines of real, over-a-coffee-table conversation.

In the virtual world, these shackles of social convention are never even a consideration; we are all there to discuss our infertility, and we can discuss it for as long as we want, in as much detail as we want, and without ever needing to apologise and feign an interest in anything else that might be happening in other people's lives or the wider world.

Through the forum I've met women whose back stories I don't even want to believe; women who've endured stillbirths, multiple miscarriages, invasive surgeries and ten years of failed treatments; women who sometimes make me feel gratitude for the relatively uneventful years of crap I myself have chalked up.

By sharing my story with these Tarantino buddies, I've discovered that everything that has, or hasn't, happened to me, will have happened, or not happened, to somebody else.

The forum, I have many times explained to DH, is the one place on earth where I can feel normal and like I belong.

Well...except, of course, for those occasions when it starts to twist into something competitive, unhealthy and sour.

You see, the trouble with being in exactly the same boat as a handful of your fellow humans is that you can't help but compare your situations. And this is exactly how the milk of human kindness we so generously pour upon one another can eventually start to curdle.

My Tarantino buddies and I share updates on the growth of

our follicles, the thickness of our womb linings, the numbers of eggs we have retrieved, the percentage that fertilise the following day, the grading of the embryos produced, the number and quality of those transferred, and the chances of success that our consultants are predicting.

And we exchange and absorb all this information, knowing that it's bound to provoke untold levels of neurosis if others around us are getting more eggs, better embryos and higher predicted odds on a successful outcome than we are.

Of course, now that I'm in the midst of my third treatment, I've learnt that it barely matters what happens before we get to the end of these two weeks. It feels like it matters enormously at the time: the scans, the numbers and the grading – but it doesn't matter at all. The only thing that matters is the end result, and after that the rest of it simply melts away into insignificance.

DH and I have had 'pretty good' everything during all of our cycles, but without the resulting pregnancy, there is no consolation prize for clearing those earlier hurdles.

In the future when people ask me whether or not we have any children, what will I tell them? 'No, but you know we *did* have some really rather promising attempts at IVF a few years back'?

Similarly, of the many, many women I've known who did indeed go on to get pregnant from extremely unpromising cycles, how many of them will answer the same question by saying, 'Oh yes, we do have children, but to be honest they appeared to be very poor quality for the couple of days they spent in a petri dish at the very start of their lives'?

I remember being overtaken by sheer disbelief at the end of our first treatment. 'But I've been through so much and we did so well!' I wanted to scream. 'Don't we get to be at least a little bit pregnant or something?'

No, we didn't, it emerged. It was simply a case of accepting that our journey had taken us right back to square one and we would now be required to do it all again, and then restart and repeat, ad tedium.

And it came as a shock to me to discover just how divisive to the forum the final results could be.

For weeks on end, my Tarantino buddies and I had stuck together like glue, acting as each other's cheerleaders when we were too defeated to cheer for ourselves. And then at the end of it all we were ruthlessly split down the middle and flung into two contrasting camps.

It's not that we weren't genuinely happy for those who had been rewarded with success. After all, we were all of us unlucky, we'd all endured so much; nobody could say that we didn't all deserve a reward for our efforts, our longed-for happy ending.

It's just that when we joined the forum we entered into a strange kind of private club, united against the cruel fertile world around us, and for the first time we each felt we could trust the other members not to betray us and to be as utterly hopeless at getting pregnant as we were.

And so it comes as a cruel blow when, at the end of this process, a select few from our gang get to wave a cheery goodbye and skip off to join another, more popular group where they'll be swapping stories about pregnancy symptoms, scans and due dates.

The betrayal by a fellow club member is even more brutal than a betrayal from the outside world, because when even the other women who could never get pregnant somehow *do*, it reveals your club as the one that nobody would ever join out of choice, and you as the queen of all losers.

This time around I already know that as I, Goldilocks, Snow, Ariel, Piglet and the other sixteen women in our online support group grind to the end of this long two-week wait, and we think about who amongst us will be pregnant at the end of it, we'll all be sharing the same irrepressible thought: I hope more than anything that it can be everyone in our group, and if there is any justice in the world then surely this will be the case. But if it turns out that it can't be, that on this occasion it will be solely just the one, well then I just hope to god in heaven that this time it's going to be me.

10.30pm

'Thanks for putting yourself through all this crap again,' DH called after me tonight, as I padded off to the bedroom in an attempt to get an early night.

He's been out fixing his bike for the best part of the day, while I've been glued to my laptop and, importantly, the latest instalments from my online friends.

I guess that some people might find the distance between us a little strange, might expect us to be inseparable for the duration of these two weeks. But we've tried the 'inseparable' approach before, and the resulting tension only makes us want to kill one another as we wait for the life-changing moment that persistently fails to materialise.

So now we simply try to mention the embryos as little as possible, as though maybe if we can convince them our backs are truly turned and the neighbourhood watch is taking a nap, they might just be tempted to break into the house that could offer them full bed and board for the next nine months.

'Well, it's something to do, isn't it?' I replied.

'It *is* something to do,' DH smiled. 'Without IVF our lives would be completely empty, wouldn't they?'

I laughed half-heartedly as I disappeared into the bedroom

and lay down carefully on my left-hand side (the sleeping position most conducive to implantation – or so I've read.)

It might be funny if it weren't so tragically true.

11.35pm

Together with Goldilocks, Snow and my other online buddies, I've created a spreadsheet, with columns to track every detail of this treatment. Each column except for the very last one is now complete: we've entered all the drug dosages, retrieval dates and numbers of embryos transferred and frozen. It's only the final outcome that remains to be revealed.

Of course, our embryos, buried deep within our bellies, will by now already know whether they're planning to implant or not, but unfortunately it will be at least another week before any of us is let in on the secret.

We'll record the results with a simple three letters as they eventually come rolling in: either BFN (Big Fat Negative) or, the most elusive sequence of letters in the alphabet for many of us, BFP (Big Fat Positive).

Tonight I've been staring at that end column with an indescribable sense of dread. In nine days' time, the box in that final column that runs parallel to my name (which, incidentally, is Genie) will contain three little letters. And the third of those three little letters is going to dictate the course of the rest of my life.

Oh, how I wish the knowledge of this filled me with excitement and hope, rather than only nausea and despair. But at least thinking about the gravity of this situation has made me realise how badly I need real friends to surround me, to support me through whatever is to come.

And so, I have finally replied to Nat and told her I'd love her to come and stay with me for a few days.

Now that the decision is made, there is, unexpectedly, a tiny part of me that is strangely looking forward to seeing this glowing and heavily pregnant friend in a couple of days' time.

I am hoping that this heavily pregnant friend of mine can start to flesh out my cardboard cut-out frame and shake me back into a three-dimensional state once again. And, ironic though it may be, I am hoping that some quality time in this pregnant friend's good company can help to remind me that there's more to this life – to any human life – than the innate ability to reproduce.

Day Seven — Monday 6th February

Sweet Dreams are Made of These

Symptoms: A few mild cramps (if I'm honest, very similar to the ones I've experienced since *before* Kenneth and Donaghy were transferred) and swollen boobs – all of which simply means that the effects of those pessaries and suppositories I'm using are undeniably kicking in now.

Hours until testing: 192

Waking hours until testing: 128

Predicted odds on this working: 7.5/10

9.20am

Waves of excitement keep washing over me this morning, and the feeling has kind of taken me by surprise after yesterday's negativity.

Instead of trying to keep my feet firmly on the ground and my imagination in check, I have today granted myself carte blanche to mentally play out the scenario where I take a positive pregnancy test in eight days' time. This time I've taken the fantasy much further than imagining when I'll take the test, how I'll tell DH, where we'll tell our mothers and if we'll immediately share the news with all our friends. This time I've worried about all the logistical elements, such as where in our highly impractical two-bedroomed flat we'll actually put our babies and all their paraphernalia once they're born, and how I'll get down our narrow communal staircase with two babies and a double buggy in tow.

Thanks to the adverse weather conditions outside, DH has been granted a surprise day off work and, true to his usual form, he has wasted no time in jumping on board and joining me in my unlikely daydream. Which means the two of us have been sitting side by side all morning, happily scouring every parenting website that exists, searching for the latest deals on prams and pushchairs, Moses baskets and nursery furniture. On the one hand, it feels like a highly premature (and some might even say *masochistic)* thing to be doing – and that's because it *is* a highly premature, and probably even a masochistic, thing to be doing. But on the other hand, if we can't get excited about these things now, then when can we?

We are both bored to death of being sensible, exercising caution and feeling too scared to enjoy even the prospect of becoming parents. It's time we had a little fun. And it genuinely *has* been fun, hunting for the best deals, and debating all the important issues, like which colour we'll paint the nursery and what kind of travel system we think would be best value for money. After an hour spent online we think we've pretty much nailed all the must-have items, and we're amazed at how inexpensive it all is. Well, considerably less expensive than IVF treatment, that's for sure.

It makes me wonder what all the parents we know have been moaning about with regards to their finances. To hear them talk, they know all about the crippling and ever-escalating costs associated with having children. But I'd like to point out to them what a sale-of-the-century bargain they've actually managed to snap up.

I'd like to inform them that DH and I currently have a down payment of around £30,000 on our children, and five years on since we placed the order and paid our first instalment, we're still waiting for them to be delivered. You don't get much shittier value than that, do you?

*

Once DH and I had finished our hypothetical shopping excursion, he jumped up and told me he'd make a start on lunch, while I sat for a moment and imagined what all the bona fide mothers might be doing with their mornings. I pictured them all out there: make-up-less and welly-clad, negotiating with tantrum-throwing toddlers, changing nappies and clearing up food and vomit and paint spillages, before necking crazy amounts of caffeine and nattering to all the other mothers they meet about teething, disrupted sleep patterns and how their ironing piles will soon be demanding a dedicated room all to themselves (although my own ironing pile is precisely this bad, and I can't even plead motherhood in my defence).

As this lucky majority stumble and fall through their chaotic days, I don't suppose many of them will pause to appreciate how fortunate they really are, and what a privilege it is to be experiencing first-hand the very unique highs and lows of parenthood. *And* that somebody not too far away would do anything in the whole world to trade places with them and to be walking in their very unglamorous and mud-encrusted wellies today.

12.00pm

Sadly, even the adverse weather conditions cannot prevent me from walking one hundred feet to the charity shop this afternoon, which means it is once again time for me to give generously to the world in this voluntary role I've chosen and to return home in a few hours, ignited by the warm glow that can only be attained through truly altruistic acts of humanity. Or, at least, that's how I packaged up this idea and sold it to myself six months ago.

6.00pm

On my way to Carol's shop this afternoon, as I trudged through the now grey and slushy snowfall, I realised how deeply worrying it is that DH and I have decided to sod waiting for the positive pregnancy test and simply go out there and start preparing everything we need for our babies' arrival. It goes against everything we were taught as children about not counting our chickens before they hatched, and it's pretty obvious that we're setting ourselves up for one almighty fall.

I also acknowledged how disturbing it might be that I've started to separate baby-related activities from actually being pregnant, and that mentally I've already begun decorating our spare bedroom as a nursery and taking my pram for strolls in the park – almost regardless of whether or not it actually contains a baby.

If this cycle doesn't end in a pregnancy, will we be the couple seen taking their greyhound and their Jack Russell into town every day, strapped in to either end of their twin buggy?

Or worse, am I eventually going to become the infertile female equivalent of Norman Bates and be discovered with scary doll babies in cribs all over my secret nursery, and terrifying family portraits of me with my doll babies framed all over our walls?

No, DH would not allow it to come to that. He'd step in, try to reason with me, encourage me to be satisfied with dressing up the greyhound in a pink bonnet and little felt booties. He'd force me to stop short of enrolling it in pre-school or attempting to breastfeed it on public transport.

Upon my arrival at the shop, I was immediately greeted by the unwelcome news that my Monday afternoon companion would be…for the second time in a week…(drum roll)…yep, you guessed it, Sylvie.

Why has this appalling example of a human being been sent to plague me during my time of greatest angst?

It's because Carol has been struck down by seasonal flu, apparently, but I can't help feeling there's some kind of sinister planetary force at work here.

'Oooh, I wanted to tell you something,' Sylvie exclaimed as I stood making us both a cup of tea in the shop's freezing, dilapidated, tiled-in-the-style-of-an-old-urinal kitchen. She tried to slip the statement in casually, as though the idea had only that second struck her, when it was patently obvious she'd been itching to collar me and tell me whatever it was from the moment I arrived.

'What's that, then?' social convention compelled me to ask, albeit through audibly gritted teeth.

She leaned in towards me, forcing me to inhale her distinctive personal aroma of stale custard creams, potpourri and hairspray, before whispering, conspiratorially, 'My friend Pat was telling me at the weekend all about her daughter Stephanie and it turns out she's had all sorts of problems in your department. Do you know, she only used to have two periods a year, poor thing? Don't know if they ever did get to the bottom of it, but the doctor put her on these tablets…can't remember what they were called…'

'Clomid?' I offered, without missing a beat.

'Yes! Clomid, that's right. And bam! Two months later she'd fallen pregnant with her little girl.'

Sylvie stood back, wide-eyed, presumably waiting for me to beg her for the contact details of her friend Pat's daughter, in the hope that I might be able to procure some of this miracle drug for myself.

'Well, that's wonderful news for Stephanie,' I told her, pinching the back of my hand to prevent myself from exploding. 'I'm glad it was so straightforward for her.'

Of course, I wasn't remotely glad for Stephanie or for her success with the most rudimentary of fertility tools. Bloody stupid Stephanie didn't realise she was born, quite frankly.

Sylvie seemed more than a little deflated; this clearly wasn't the reaction she'd anticipated.

'It's amazing really what they can do today, isn't it?' she continued, determined to keep the conversation going one way or another.

'Yes, science is moving forward all the time,' I agreed, not a trace of a smile on my face. 'Doctors can help a lot more people these days.'

'Hmmmm,' she murmured, her insipid, blue-veined hand now pawing at my sleeve. 'But the important thing is not to give up, dear. Because it *will* happen when…you know, when you've forgotten about it and decided to…do something else.'

Forgotten about it, ha! How many more times am I going to hear that one before I can't nod and smile any longer? Before I'm forced to point out the unwitting idiocy of these people who tell you it will only happen when you've given up entirely – and then tell you to take comfort in that knowledge and remember never to give up?

'Yes,' I told her, exercising great restraint not to smash a heavy object over her head, 'that's why I've decided to just not think about it anymore and to leave it all in God's capable hands.'

Sylvie simply nodded her head approvingly at this point, while I resolved to bring God into all future conversations of this nature. Whatever the beliefs of those involved, his appearance does seem to bring an abrupt ending to the discussion – an ending for which I can only feel religiously grateful.

Trekking back home through the sludge after my shift had finished, I thought more carefully about Sylvie's words, and concluded that at least one statement to leave her mouth this afternoon had been correct: there really are incredible things that doctors can do today. But what I didn't share with her is what it feels like when you realise that, for you personally, not even one of these incredible medical breakthroughs will actually fucking well work.

7.30pm

DH is in the kitchen putting the finishing touches on his homemade pizza, and I've been instructed to 'put my feet up with a cuppa' for the next half hour.

There should be something kind of validating about being the one to arrive home from work and walking into a light, warm flat and a spouse preparing dinner; it should make me feel as though I'm contributing to our little household again, but today it only makes me feel even more pathetic than I did when I was living as a totally unemployed hermit.

At least back then I could claim I was being true to myself in some way.

'Good day in the office?' DH asked when I walked through the door.

'Don't. I'm not in the mood,' I snapped at him. 'I know it's not a proper job. I know I'm a fucking failure. I have no idea what I'm supposed to be doing with my life anymore.'

And with that, I burst into tears; no warning, no provocation, just full-on, snot-spraying, body-shaking sobbing that caught both of us completely unawares.

DH rushed over to put his arms around me, his hands still covered in various pizza toppings, no doubt wondering what on earth he'd said or done that was so terribly wrong this time.

'I just wish I knew what I'd done to deserve this,' I managed to choke out between desperate gulps for air.

'You didn't *do* anything,' DH tried to assure me, as he placed his hands on my shoulders and forced me to look him in the eye.

'Life's just shit sometimes, that's all,' he said, with a prevailing smile and a shrug.

But I told him I couldn't accept that argument; insisted that I must have done *something*, must have made some unforgivable error along the way to deserve this cross that the two of us now bear.

DH laughed and suggested that maybe it was just because I had always refused to eat my greens as a kid.

'But maybe it really *is* something that stupid,' I continued, thinking of all the other dietary sins I've committed over the years that may have rendered me infertile.

Or maybe this misfortune has been dished out as some form of punishment, because I once two-timed a boyfriend for the space of about a week, or because I took poppers with my friend Hannah in a dance tent in Glastonbury during the summer of 1994.

Or perhaps I'm not being punished by a higher power, and it's simply the fact that my body aged irrevocably during the year of the 'horrible boss' at work, which was also the year when my teammates buggered off on maternity leave or emigrated with their boyfriends and left me drinking turbo-strength coffee and going boss-eyed in front of my computer screen until 10.00pm every night.

No matter what the reason, our present situation leads me to one definite conclusion: 'We should've started trying *years* ago,' I told DH, bitterly.

'We did!' he laughed.

'No, I mean years and years ago,' I snapped. 'I should've started trying when I was sixteen.'

'Er…who with?' DH asked, with great curiosity.

'ANYONE!' I shouted.

DH raised his eyebrows and started to shake his head. 'Obviously I didn't mean that,' I added quickly, immediately aware that I had totally overstepped the mark this time.

And obviously I didn't *mean* it – but it didn't stop me from *thinking* it from time to time.

I mean, sure, having a baby at sixteen would've stopped me from going to university, stopped me from travelling, stopped me from meeting DH, even. But maybe, just maybe, had I spent my youth indiscriminately shagging as many virile people of the opposite sex as I could possibly get my hands on, maybe I would at least by now be a mother.

Granted, I'd probably also be the proud owner of every STD under the sun, but I wonder how that alternate life – of single, syphilis-riddled mother – would compare to the one I'm living right now.

I suppose what I'm really asking is whether a single, syphilis-riddled mother could possibly feel any unhappier than I do at this point in time.

'I just wish I was younger,' I explained to DH, miserably, a little later on.

And that really *is* the bottom line here. From this day forward, all I know for certain is that there won't be a single day that passes me by where I won't wish that I was five years, three years or even just *one* year younger than I am today. Just so that I would have a little more time, so I might feel I had a little more chance of winning this race against my biological clock.

9.45pm

As we sat eating our pizza this evening, I presented DH with the possibility that we could, reliably, test a couple of days before our official test date in eight days' time – or, less reliably, even a couple of days from now.

I told him about some of my Tarantino buddies, Goldilocks, Piglet and Snow, who are just a couple of days ahead of me in their two-week waits and who have already given in to the temptation of the home pregnancy test – with, I've been forced to admit, somewhat mixed results.

Piglet and Snow have been greeted by the faint emergence of

a second line – the very early BFP – and so can now, albeit cautiously, breathe a massive sigh of relief and start to enjoy the first flutters of genuine excitement. I can see that they have done themselves a gigantic favour and can now face their remaining days with a real sense of hope and optimism.

In fact, reading their posts has made me want to tear into our spare bedroom, wrench out that stiff bottom drawer and pee on every single pregnancy stick that I've been stashing away for our official test date on Valentine's Day.

But I must pause to consider both eventualities here. After all, there are other online buddies, Goldilocks included, who have also succumbed to the lure of the early test and who have, as a result, been faced with the all-consuming horror that is the BFN.

Straightaway, DH's hackles rose when I mentioned first the prospect of the early testing and then the forbidden forum, and he curtly dismissed the topic by telling me that we *would* be following our crystal-clear instructions from the clinic and we *would* be waiting for our scheduled test date, as previously agreed.

I wish it was a little easier to talk to him about all this stuff. And I wish I could share his certainty that simply waiting obediently for another eight days is the kindest, the sanest, and the most sensible thing to do.

I remember very clearly that I *did* share his certainty during our first cycle. I knew then that if I had to see a BFN, then at the very least I had to be able to trust it, because there was no way in hell that I could bear to see something so terrible twice.

I remember that I had even begun to worry, as our official test date loomed, that I would never have the guts to take the test, that I would reach and surpass our official date without summoning the courage to find out.

But of course, I needn't have worried. Because the torture of not knowing, in the end, outweighed even the agony of a potentially negative result.

And once I was holding that negative result in my hand, I couldn't forgive myself for waiting so long, for allowing myself to carry around all that false hope for fourteen whole days.

Around nine months later, as we prepared for the final two weeks in our second IVF cycle, I vowed that I would not be making the same mistake again. That time, I promised myself that I would take control of the situation, I would demand to know what was going on inside my body; goddammit, I would test every single day until that elusive second line began to surface if that's what it took.

It seemed like a sensible strategy at the time. But as the first five mornings' test results rolled in and the single lines continued to brazenly emerge, I began to realise that my foolproof plan had been horribly naive.

Although I kept telling myself (and DH) that our second cycle *had* to have worked, I could already sense that there wouldn't be a pregnancy test on the planet that was going to agree.

I realise now, as I commit this to paper, that I must have sounded like a raving lunatic, but since history suggested that the pregnancy tests would always work against me, I felt sure that my only chance of a successful outcome was to try a different approach.

And so over to the clinic we drove to ask a nurse to stick a needle in my vein and measure the level of HCG in my blood.

I remember explaining to our nurse, a matronly, slightly stern woman called Joanna, that I was feeling 'worryingly normal' when she asked how I was doing. But Joanna simply shrugged and tried to reassure me that women in my position are frequently convinced that nothing has happened, when in fact their bodies have been calmly getting on with the task of becoming pregnant the whole time, just without the sort of fanfare we might have come to expect.

But somehow, as I sat in that chair and watched the crimson red liquid flowing from my open vein into a small test tube, I knew beyond a shadow of doubt that there would be no happy, surprise-of-our-lives revelation waiting in store for us.

Back at home a few hours later, we contemplated not bothering to pick up the phone when Joanna called with our results, knowing what she was going to say before the words had formed in her mouth.

'I'm afraid it's not good news,' she told DH, a hint of sadness cutting into her usual matter-of-fact tone.

'It's okay, we know,' DH told her, his hand searching for mine and squeezing it tightly as he spoke.

'You know?' she asked, confused.

'Sometimes you just know,' he had explained, before gently ending the call.

It was the truth. Sometimes you really do just know. And surprise, surprise, it really wasn't any easier having the devastating news delivered by a virtual stranger. In fact, if anything, driving to the clinic to take the test and seeing all the staff again made it somehow even more awful.

As DH placed his phone back on the coffee table, we simply stared at one another, wordlessly acknowledging that maybe there had been a tiny fragment of hope alive in us after all – but that it had just now been ruthlessly butchered to death before our eyes.

I took a few moments to honour the build-up over the last three months: the special sperm- and egg-priming diets we'd obeyed, the exercising, the fertility yoga, the acupuncture, the teetotalism, the social hibernation, the injections, the medical procedures, the meditation, the anxiety, the hope, the £6,500 we'd scraped together over the last nine months to spend on this supposedly life-altering treatment – all culminating in the apologetic two-minute phone call we'd just received.

I could see from DH's pained expression that similar thoughts were tumbling through his mind.

'Right, well that's that then,' he'd said, eventually, placing his hand on my knee.

'Yes,' I agreed, after a brief pause. 'As we were, then.'

And with that, DH dragged himself up from the sofa and went to stick the kettle on for a cup of tea.

We knew the drill by that stage. We knew the last few months had been nothing but a private nightmare the two of us had shared, and that there was nothing for it but to place the needle back on the record and pick up where we'd left off.

Except that I couldn't do it that time. Unlike our first failed cycle, where I'd been left feeling guilty, ashamed and like I'd let the whole team down, this time I was simply incandescent with rage.

I was suddenly so overwhelmed with anger that I didn't dare attend our review meeting until a whole month had passed. Had I gone sooner, I feared I might have grabbed Dr Kapoor, our consultant, by the scruff of his neck and demanded that he explain why he had done this to us – or just skipped the small talk and put him straight through the nearest window.

Would we like to make use of the free counselling service, I knew he would ask. No, we did NOT want a fucking counselling session, I felt like screaming in anticipation of his ludicrous question. We wanted the free early pregnancy scan that was also part of our pre-paid IVF package. I wanted our embryos back, I wanted them growing inside me, I wanted the baby that he had led us to believe would be waiting for us at the end of this twisted game.

Not that he had led us to believe that we would be taking home a baby, of course.

It's a popular belief that doctors like Dr Kapoor prey upon the infertile, luring us into their clinics with promises of guaranteed treatments and happy-ever-afters.

In reality, they are not guilty of this crime. Such is the power of infertility and our desire to escape its clutches that consultants need never lie to us at all; instead, they can just tell us gravely that there is around a seventy per cent chance that we are throwing our money, our mental health, our emotional well-being and a substantial portion of our lives down the toilet in pursuit of this wild goose, and then watch as we tear the consent forms out of their hands to sign up for the next chase.

Dr Kapoor himself had basically implied that he thought we were all maniacs, that he himself would never dream of entering into such an absurd lottery.

Rationally, I knew I had no right to hurl him through the window of his office. But being reasonable and rational in this type of situation is wholly unsatisfying. Both DH and I were in need of someone to blame and a bald-headed fertility doctor to disembowel.

I wonder if perhaps this is why DH is so reluctant to discover the final result this time. We both know there is nobody left to blame and no explanation left to offer when life delivers these blows.

So, in his own uncommunicative way, I think DH is simply making it known that he would prefer to drift within the bubble of possibility for a little longer, if that's quite alright with me.

And, after all he has endured these past few years, who the hell am I to threaten to stick a pin in that precious bubble tonight?

Day Eight – Tuesday 7th February

A Fat Friend Comes to Stay

Symptoms: Sore boobs (nothing special about that at this stage in an IVF, or even a natural, cycle), a rather attractive boil on my right temple, and a strange pimple on the skin below my right thumbnail. Sadly, an extensive trawl of the Internet reveals neither of the latter two ailments to be a positive indication of pregnancy.

Hours until testing: 168

Waking hours until testing: 112

Predicted odds on this working: 5/10

11.00am

The snow of the last few days has mostly melted, DH has been forced to return to work, and I think I might have officially entered purgatory.

Since waking from a fitful sleep at 6.00am, I've been searching for things to calm my jangling nerves, and for the last few hours have resorted to listening to online interviews with inspirational businesswomen from around the world.

Like every other distraction technique I've tried to date, it hasn't helped in the slightest. Most of the interviewees find themselves choked with emotion when asked about their children and the transformative role they've played within their lives. And the miniscule handful who haven't produced offspring themselves simply leave me in awe of their achievements and wondering what the fuck I've been doing with my thirty-five years on this earth.

One of these interviewees was even honest enough to confess that she'd willingly trade in her multi-million-pound business empire for the family she'd always dreamed about but never managed to create. It was not what I'd wanted to hear. Because if even this woman can't find happiness and fulfilment in spite of her phenomenal success, then what hope is there for somebody like me?

Before he left for work earlier, DH asked me what Nat and I might like to do when he returns home this evening – and I'm afraid I'm feeling quite stuck for ideas.

It's difficult to explain to other people that, to be truthful, I don't want to go out, I don't want to stay in, I don't want to speak to anyone, I don't want to be left alone, I don't want to talk about anything to do with my possibly pregnant state, and yet, in spite this, I can think of ABSOLUTELY NOTHING ELSE.

I appreciate that this does not make me the easiest person to help, entertain or generally be around – and that I'll be burdening not only DH but also my best friend with this impossible task for the next couple of days.

Perhaps my invitation to Nat should have come with a little more of a warning?

11.55am

Kenneth and Donaghy are now eight days old, and I've been anxiously reading about how their short lives should so far be progressing.

If they are destined to become our babies, then they will already have attached to my uterine lining and burrowed into my womb. If they haven't done this by now…well, then, their tiny flickering lights will already have been extinguished.

The one remaining pragmatic splinter of my brain is urging me to think like Dr Rangan, to view this strange baby-making process as a coin toss or a game of rock, paper, scissors – get the result you don't want and it's all okay, because you simply keep moving the goalposts: best of three, best of five, best of seven, best of ten. We've all heard tales of the woman who got pregnant on her fifteenth IVF attempt; it's just a case of never giving up, never taking a BFN for a final answer (including from your bank manager), and furiously pursuing this one target no matter what the sacrifices, no matter what the cost.

But it's hard to be pragmatic when it's your heart and soul, as well as your time and bank balance, that you've invested in this gamble.

And I suspect there's probably a pretty good reason why you don't come across too many couples who've been through fifteen rounds of IVF.

12.30pm

There are five hours to kill before I need to collect Nat from the coach station, and I need to somehow force myself into a more positive mindset before she arrives.

It would really help if I could take a little mental holiday from this torture and pass the responsibility of trying to get pregnant on to somebody else for a while. Ideally, I'd like to hire some kind of private fertility detective, who would turn up in a raincoat, headscarf and dark glasses, remove the problem from my hands and make it her personal mission to get us our baby. She'd leave no stone unturned in her quest to figure out what the source of our problem was, and then she'd fix it and turn up at a carefully selected location, brown envelope in hand.

She'd push it across the table towards us, lean in and whisper that it was okay, we were pregnant now, and the envelope contained all the scan photos we'd need to prove that our baby really would be here now in a few months and all would be well.

Failing that, it would be helpful if I could allocate a few days of my two-week wait to DH or one of my friends, just so they could relieve me of the anguish of wondering whether I'm pregnant or not during every single minute of every hour of every day.

Even over the course of this morning I've found myself lifting up my jumper and peering down suspiciously at my belly. I do hope you're looking after things in there, I think worriedly.

I've also spent a good ten minutes in front of the bathroom mirror, performing an in-depth nipple investigation for what must have been the hundredth time to date. My objective, as ever, was to hunt for positive, pregnancy-affirming evidence, perhaps in the form of a slight pigmentation change or a prominent blue vein or two beginning to surface beneath the top layer of skin. Even the most thorough inspection reveals no real difference, of course, but I know that won't stop me from getting my nipples out for analysis at least another three hundred times before this two-week wait is over.

I honestly don't know why I pay them this sort of attention anymore. One thing I've learnt over the years is that my boobs cannot be trusted to provide solid evidence of a pregnancy any more than they could be trusted to complete a Sudoku puzzle or parallel park. They are rotten liars, teasers and pranksters, the pair of them. And they are even audaciously sitting here now, swollen, painful, itchy and screaming out to me that they are eagerly preparing for their first stint as milk machines, when I know for a fact that they've been acting like this since before an embryo was within a hundred yards of my body.

Oh, lord, how sickeningly familiar this is all starting to feel. And how desperately I want to feel something different; just something – anything – I haven't felt already a hundred times before.

7.30pm

Well, Nat is now here – in our flat, pregnant and curled up quite comfortably on our sofa.

In the car on the way back from the coach station she was chatting away, telling me how much she was looking forward to a few days' break from her three-year-old son, so she could focus her flagging energy supply on the nice, quiet, compliant baby in her belly and on simply being herself.

I wish I could focus on the nice, quiet almost-babies in my belly and enjoy simply being myself, too. But to be honest I think I'd rather be anything other than myself right now.

Around half an hour ago, Nat and I stood side by side in the kitchen and lined up all our prenatal multivitamins and supplements along the counter, as though we were just like any other expectant friends, happily hanging out together and nurturing their blossoming bumps.

But the truth is that only Nat qualifies for the pregnant club right now, while I am simply tagging along in her shadow – and feeling like an absolute fraud.

Within less than ten minutes of her arrival, I had confided in Nat (well, more like blurted it out in the middle of a totally unrelated conversation) that we were coming to the end of yet another IVF cycle.

A huge part of me wanted to keep these cards close to my chest, but what I'm going through right now is just too huge, too scary, too all-consuming. And God it felt good to actually talk about it and get at least some of the worry out in the open. I know I'll probably live to regret it, but at least now I have a justified reason to share the repetitive contents of my head and to interrupt every conversation after thirty seconds so that I can wonder aloud whether or not I might finally be pregnant, because I have to be, don't I? And then to confess that I'm shaken to the core by the fear that I won't be. And then to explain how badly I need to believe this time that I will be. And then to reveal that I just *know* deep down that I won't be. And then to pose the question that I *must* be this time…mustn't I?

To her great credit, Nat has graciously indulged this endless rambling and questioning and has assured me, several times, that she did not experience any pregnancy symptoms whatsoever in either of her pregnancies until long after her period was missed. There was no implantation bleeding, no implantation pain, no frequent urination, no metallic tastes and no morning sickness.

Her only clue, she promises me (in fact swears to me, on her life), was slightly swollen boobs, and I am so very grateful to her for telling me this that I have made her repeat it at least fifty times this evening, and will make her repeat it at least another hundred times before she returns home in two days' time.

10.30pm

Looking back on it, this day can only be described as a bittersweet experience, and it has just ended with something completely unexpected, something I have never before observed. I've known for a while now that DH is accomplished at hiding his true feelings, that he could even be described as the master of reserve. But for those first few seconds when he arrived home this evening and walked over to greet our friend, he couldn't quite mask his discomfort or his disgust at the bump that so proudly protruded from beneath her fluffy winter pyjamas.

I, of course, had been trying to pre-empt and prepare myself for this devastating vision, and had already taken the decision that I would be regarding Nat as nothing more than a floating head and shoulders for the duration of her stay. But DH had not prepared himself at all, and suddenly there it was, confronting him, this symbol of everything he had worked so hard for and was still being denied; this most wonderfully womanly gift that his poor, broken wife just could not seem to deliver.

The barely detectable revulsion flashed across his face in a matter of seconds, but I had caught it there as plain as day, loyally protecting my damaged heart, assuring me that he was not in any way impressed by or in awe of this other, more reproductively capable creature who was sat next to me on our sofa, unavoidably highlighting my defectiveness.

I couldn't be sure whether or not Nat had also caught this fleeting glimpse into DH's psyche, although by the way she shifted uncomfortably in her seat and drew her pyjamas tightly around her, I would guess that maybe she had.

I feel genuinely sorry for any awkwardness or shame she might have felt in that moment, because she has done absolutely nothing to warrant any feelings of guilt.

But seeing that look on my husband's face tonight has been worth more than a thousand words. It has made me realise how destructive to him this ordeal really is, and how little of his suffering I get to see each day.

It has also reignited my love for the man with a ferocity I can't recall feeling before now.

Day Nine — Wednesday 8th February

A Woman's Worst Nightmare

Symptoms: None. Just the overwhelming urge to break down and cry. I've come to the conclusion that, when it comes to symptoms, *something*, in fact *anything*, is better than nothing. It's our bodies eerily ticking along as though nothing is happening that strikes fear into our hearts. And it's because it makes us fear precisely that: that NOTHING is happening.

Hours remaining: 144

Waking hours remaining: 96

Predicted odds on this working: 2/10

8.45am

'The fear' has officially sunk its talons into either side of my head and is refusing to let go. Never mind chasing after the coattails of the glowing positivity I felt the other day; today I cannot even find the trail of dust it left behind.

I know the dark feelings I'm experiencing will not be helped by the fact that I took a pregnancy test thirty minutes ago — and it was, of course, negative.

I think I took the test at this incredibly early stage because I knew deep down that it was definitely too early to get an accurate result. I hoped that by some miracle the stick might show me the very first beginnings of a second line, but I comforted myself with the knowledge that if it didn't it would still be okay, because there really should be nothing to see at this point.

It didn't stop me from staring at the damned thing at regular intervals for more than half an hour, though.

I can vaguely remember reading online personal accounts of pregnancy tests that have taken five or ten minutes to develop an accurate result. And as I sat staring at my stick, I was tempted to post the desperate question to my Tarantino buddies: 'What's the longest length of time a pregnancy test can take to give you a positive result?'

Could it be one hour? Several days? Could it be nine months?

Of course it can't be, but that won't stop me from digging that ridiculous stick out of the bin to scrutinise it every time I pass the bedroom for the rest of the day. Christ, I've even been known to forage through bin liners to unearth negative pregnancy tests that I felt certain must have transformed into positives the moment they believed my back was turned.

I wonder if it's only the negative pregnancy test that's making my nerve endings feel so alive today, or whether it's maternal instinct kicking in, telling me that, just like last time and the time before, our embryos are no longer in this race.

Or maybe I'm just more on edge today because a heavily pregnant Nat is still enjoying a much-needed lie-in in the spare room, and because I'm so impatient to jump off this hostile island where I've been marooned for the last five years and join her on the rich and bountiful mainland.

Part of me questions my motives for having Nat here to stay at this god-awful time, and I wonder if, by having her here, I'm trying to activate Karma in some way.

'Look over here,' I seem to be yelling. 'Watch me embracing somebody else's pregnancy joy in the most difficult of personal circumstances! Behold my selflessness as I try to ignore my own hardships for the sake of somebody else!'

Could Mother Nature be so cruel as to deny me once again after going through all of this turmoil?

I'm not even sure I want to find out.

DH pointed out to me recently, in one of his rarer moments of empathy, that it's understandable why I feel the way I do sometimes, since I'm currently realising what has to be most women's number one nightmare.

And it's true that if a woman is involved in an accident, gets diagnosed with a serious illness, or has to undergo some kind of surgery, the first question past her lips, often before, 'Am I going to die?' is, 'Am I still going to be able to have children?'

I know it would be the first question that would occur to me. But I feel terrible admitting that. Because bad things, very bad things, are happening to other people right now. There are other agonising two-week waits in this life. Like the wait to see if your latest cancer treatment will be successful (and my dad, like so many others, knew all about that one). So what gives me the right to hold infertility up as the worst thing that could ever happen? After all, I am not dying, am I?

Although, in a small but significant way, maybe I am. You see, infertility robs you of your genetic link to the future, reminds you of your mortality, plants in the forefront of your brain all those unanswerable questions, like why am I here? What's the meaning of it all? What will I leave behind?

And, sure enough, when the reality of the situation hits, it'll leave you screaming in its wake, 'NO! Not me! Not this! Please, I'll swap with anyone! I'll do anything! Just please don't let this be the story of *my* life.'

Had I been given a list of ten awful fates that could have

befallen me and asked to make my choice…well, I know how heinous the other nine would need to be for me to choose not being able to have children as my destiny.

And if a deal with the devil were on the table right now, I wonder what I would agree to if it meant I would be getting to meet my gorgeous, healthy bouncing baby in nine months' time. Would I trade a leg, an arm? The right to ask for anything good to happen ever again? Would I trade *other people's* legs and arms and their rights to a happy existence? I guess you can never truly know what depths you'd sink to until your back's against the wall.

11.30am

Poor Nat. I have just inflicted Bobby McFerrin's 'Don't Worry, Be Happy' upon her for the third time this morning. I don't know why I imagined this would be a good idea, because if there's one song guaranteed to make me want to cry when I'm already feeling like crap then it's probably this one.

Nat has tentatively enquired a couple of times now about how I'm feeling, and I've tried my best to answer her question, while also trying to protect her from the full contents of my head.

Having had a total absence of 'symptoms' for the last twenty-four hours, I did, around thirty minutes ago, experience a couple of sharp stomach cramps, which have simultaneously filled me with immense hope and utter despair.

I wondered if the cramps were a sign that Kenneth and Donaghy are busy implanting into my womb as we speak, or if, alternatively, they're a sign that they've stopped developing altogether and my womb is getting ready to chuck itself inside out as soon as I stop taking the pessaries in a few days' time.

Or maybe it's the pessaries themselves that are causing those brief, niggly cramps.

Or maybe the cramps are not even real; perhaps they're just a figment of my imagination, fuelled only by my desperate desire to rustle up some sort of pregnancy-confirming evidence.

In any case, having shared the condensed version of this intense inner debate with Nat, she's told me she believes the cramps must be a strongly encouraging sign that exciting things are taking place in my belly right now. Well, what else can the poor girl say?

3.30pm

Later this afternoon, Nat and I went out for a very sensible organic lunch, and she swore to me on her life for the twenty-seventh time that I *would* not and *should* not be feeling anything out of the ordinary this early on. Her only real clues, she is adamant, were still only the slightly swollen boobs, the missed period and the positive pregnancy test.

The swollen boobs and the late period are good news. I know that, with the support of the pessaries I'm using, I might just be on track for one of those. The positive test is far more troubling, however, as this is where I and all the genuinely pregnant women have dramatically parted company in the past.

While we were crunching through our broccoli and spinach salads and sipping our green teas, Nat asked me how I would feel about having twins, now that it's supposedly a very real possibility.

I could tell by the look in her eye that she didn't think I'd make it out of the first week alive if I really did give birth to two babies at the same time – but she did a good job of trying to shield me from her true opinion and told me instead that she thinks it will be a lovely outcome if indeed it comes about.

And then we went on to discuss the horrors of childbirth and the impossibility of juggling everything else in our lives with the responsibility of motherhood.

It felt good to be able to join in with the worries, excitement and trepidation of the expectant mums' club for once.

And I am so ready to cross this barrier and get on with the next challenge of actually being pregnant.

After all, it's not as if pregnancy doesn't pose its own problems, and I know that even if we do get good news in a few days' time, we're certainly not out of the woods. In fact, it would be more accurate to say that we'll have barely set foot *inside* the woods at that stage.

I think I might have said earlier in this two-week wait that I wanted someone to put me into stasis and wake me up when I was pregnant. Well, I got that very wrong.

What I really want is for someone to put me into stasis and wake me only when I've given birth to our baby. Because I know only too well that the elation of a positive pregnancy test can be ruthlessly short-lived.

The official two-week wait, once over, is immediately replaced by the agonising two- or three-week wait for the first scan, which will confirm whether or not there is a detectable heartbeat. And this is followed by another agonising wait for the all-important twelve-week scan, and then the twenty-week scan, and then the birth. And that's before you consider all the totally normal fears DH and I would have about whether we'd be able to cope with having a baby, and whether or not we'd actually be any good at it.

But that train of thought is far too depressing to share with Nat, who is sitting across from me, trying so hard to be positive and optimistic on my behalf.

And anyway, I can't expect her to ever truly understand. In amongst the pregnancy chat, she has not been able to resist the chance to talk of her longing for an escape from the humdrum nature of family life and the banality of baby talk with other new mums.

I guess this is the fantasy that consumes her mind, just as the fantasy of finally becoming pregnant will continue to consume mine.

'Look at you, you look so nice and healthy and…normal,' she told me suddenly over lunch. 'I don't know how I became so old and boring and haggard in the last couple of years.'

She told me she doesn't understand how or why she's been abruptly awoken at the age of thirty-five, when only a couple of years ago, it seems to her, the two of us were standing in each other's bedrooms debating the length of skirt you could get away with if you wore hot-pants underneath, and lounging around in cheap cafes nursing hangovers and filling in the drunken blanks to piece together the jigsaw puzzle of the previous night's escapades.

I am equally at a loss to explain the mystery of this vanishing decade. I thought I had my whole life stretching ahead of me: time to have fun, time to discover the world, even time to give up my job in a small marketing team in south London and realise my ambition of becoming a world-renowned artist.

I guess somewhere down the line I must've taken my eye off the ball. And suddenly there I was, my youth and my prime behind me, handing in a letter of resignation to my boss on a sunny Friday afternoon, with no idea of what was supposed to come next.

Unlike my friends and work colleagues, I didn't get to walk out in a blaze of glory, stepping through the giant revolving door in a sea of flowers, fond farewells and maternity vouchers as I launched myself into the next chapter of my life.

Instead, I found myself quietly slinking out the back door under a cloud of suspicion and disappointment, to pursue a future in costly medical treatments and daytime TV.

Those who knew what was going on said it was the right thing to do, and that I'd really had no choice. But I knew even at the time that it was never going to feel okay.

*

Back at the table with Nat, as I was mentally reliving the final weeks and days of my work life, I tried to concentrate on what she was telling me about her own wasted child-free years, about how she'll never now be able to muster the energy required to fulfil any of her ambitions or do anything remotely interesting with her life.

She yawned as she tugged at the loose curls escaping from her hurriedly scraped-up ponytail.

And I had to refrain from telling her that I feel exactly the same as she does. After all, I've sacrificed my career, social life and personal ambitions for my children as well. But, unlike Nat, I just haven't fucking well met mine yet.

I know I must NOT vocalise that thought.

So instead I just confessed my deepest personal regret: not starting to try for a family at least one hundred years sooner.

I admitted I hadn't realised at the time that there might be a choice to be made. It was as though I believed on some level that my children already existed, that they were dangling from some kind of cosmic washing line, just waiting for some indeterminable point in the future when I'd snap my fingers and decide the time was right to pluck them off and bring them down here into my life.

But that wasn't how it was going to work for me. And now it was all looking like a classic case of too little, too late.

'But it's just all so…predictable,' Nat proceeded to tell me as she explained how self-ravaging the rituals of her average day have become and how she's acquired a level of weariness that she knows no amount of early nights, lie-ins or under-eye cream could ever now hope to reverse.

I can't pretend to have a clue what she means, of course. I don't know what it's like to have little people shouting, 'Mummy! Mummy! MUUMMEEE!' all day long, to never be able to go for a wee on your own, to make spaghetti bolognese and then watch your dinner dates tip it straight over their heads, to stay up all night comforting a teething toddler, to spend hours coercing and pleading with very small people to put shoes and coats on so you can at last leave the fucking house.

But I *want* to know this life. Because that stuff gives you stories, first-hand experiences, and the right to exchange knowing smiles of solidarity with other frazzled parents as you all manoeuvre your wayward shopping trolleys around the aisles of Tesco.

And it comes with other stuff, too: the *good* stuff. The stuff that Nat and other kind friends will never tell me about now, for precisely that reason: they are trying to be kind. But I know that it exists: the first smiles, the contented gurgles, the laughter, the feeling of being at the centre of someone's universe, the kisses and cuddles, the sense of recognition you must feel as you look into a tiny face and discover some essence of your partner, and your brother, and your great-grandparent staring back at you.

Maybe if I promised to be the world's most patient mother, to never complain or compare, to never want or ask for another single thing for the rest of my life – would the fertility gods finally agree to give me my chance?

11.30pm

When DH arrived home tonight at around 8.30pm, the three of us took a short walk over to The Three Cups, our local pub, where a mediocre, middle-aged jazz band were playing. They were nothing to write home about, but the atmosphere was uplifting and friendly, and the roaring log fire in the corner provided some welcome warmth from the winter chill outside.

Nat attracted the usual attention that heavily pregnant women come to expect, with total strangers offering her encouraging smiles, apologising profusely for jostling her at the bar, and even stopping to ask her when she was due and whether or not she was expecting a girl or a boy.

Too late, I spotted my nemesis co-worker Sylvie dancing a kind of geriatric chicken dance in front of the stage, and before I could turn away she had caught my eye and come darting over to brag about knowing one of the backing singers from her school days. Against my better judgement, I found myself introducing her to Nat, and then in the next instant she had clocked the bump and begun interrogating my poor friend on every aspect of her pregnancy.

An uncomfortable and embarrassed Nat had turned virtually monosyllabic in response, and was doing a pretty good impression of a woman who had less interest in her current pregnancy than in the packet of salt and vinegar crisps in her hand. But then, just to complete the horrifying scene, DH had returned from the bar and Sylvie had wasted no time at all in placing one hand on Nat's bulging belly, the other on DH's arm, and congratulating him on his impending bundle of joy. Watching his baffled expression, I had leapt in to correct her that DH was in fact *my* husband, not the proud father of Nat's unborn second child.

Oblivious to the extent of her social faux pas, Sylvie simply laughed, apologised, congratulated Nat again and then danced the funky chicken all the way back to the stage. Leaving the three of us standing there, teeth clenched in a forced smile as the tumbleweed entwined our feet.

I don't know why her simple mistake had cut so deep, but it was suddenly very clear to me that, to the untrained eye, DH looked like the happy husband of a glowing soon-to-be mum. Which, if only he had chosen his life partner a little more wisely, is exactly what he would be.

It was obvious that DH and Nat were feeling similarly uncomfortable, and the pair of them just stood there, looking guilt-ridden and sheepish, as though they'd just been confronted with watertight evidence of the torrid affair they'd been conducting behind my back.

Nat pulled her coat around her bump, as though to conceal their shameful lovechild, while DH and I gulped down our drinks and stared desperately at the stage.

It seemed more than a little unfortunate that the four band members had chosen this moment to take an interval between songs, and were hanging about at the back of the pub doing nothing noteworthy whatsoever.

Around an hour later we were all more than ready to head home, and I walked out onto the street feeling like a social leper; someone who should stay within the confines of her house until she found a way to fit in with the rest of this fertile world.

As we stepped outside, a thick ground frost was forming on top of the now grey and sludgy snow from a few days ago. Even in the short time we had been inside, it had turned whole sections of the High Street into an icy death trap and, as soon as he realised the danger, DH instinctively grabbed for me, determined to prevent our embryos from being jolted out of my womb by a hefty thump to the ground.

Of course, he probably *should* have focused on helping the genuinely pregnant woman first, the one whom he left wobbling along precariously for a few brief moments until he remembered his manners and responsibilities.

But he didn't, because his gut reaction was to leave her to fall to her death and to grab for the other woman instead, the one who has been crying wolf for a full five years now.

In that split second, he revealed not what he felt he *must* or *ought* to say or do as a dutiful husband, but what he wholeheartedly *believed*.

I don't know how it's possible, but it seems that DH still holds out a little hope for a happy ending, still has a little faith that his babies are being nurtured by my body on this cold, cold night.

And this can only mean that he still holds out a little hope – *enough* hope at least – that, even after all my failures and false starts, *I* might eventually come good.

Day Ten — Thursday 9th February

The People Next Door

Symptoms: A slight pulling sensation near my left ovary, bloating and a dull headache. In summary: absolutely nothing worth mentioning at all.

Hours remaining: 120

Waking hours remaining: 80

Predicted odds on this working: 2/10

7.30am

Since DH and Nat are still asleep, I've taken the opportunity to log on to the forum and see how all my Tarantino buddies are getting on. Having a quick scan through their posts, I can see that we're divided into two distinct camps now: those who are frantically symptom-spotting and obsessing over every breath, itch and fart, and those who are just calmly riding out this inevitable wait, fully accepting that there is nothing they can do to influence the outcome either way.

Those in the first group (and I include myself in this group, of course) are deluded fools, whipping themselves into a state of false hope or needless paranoia.

And those in the second group, in my opinion at least, are the ones who, through either instinct or hard evidence, already know that their treatment has worked. Well, either that or they're just abject liars.

An early-morning post from Ariel reads: *Been feeling sick on and off for the last 24 hours and almost threw up while cooking dinner last night. Got a strange pulling sensation inside and feeling very sensitive to smells. Just don't know what to think!*

Well, Ariel may claim today that she knows not what to think, but I'm pretty sure I know what she wants us to tell her *we* think.

Sounds very encouraging, we all reply. *Probably really early morning sickness setting in and your uterus stretching to accommodate the pregnancy.*

Why do we all do this to ourselves?

I am no different, obviously.

I was trying to explain to Nat just last night that the only situation to which I can liken the two-week wait is a global 'red alert' state of biological warfare.

It's as though I sat down to eat breakfast, turned on the morning news and found every station dominated by an urgent news flash about a deadly virus which has broken out, is airborne and is currently infiltrating every home on the planet.

Ashen-faced newsreaders have gone on to explain that everyone who starts to feel nauseous in the next seventy-two hours will have a level of natural immunity to the disease and should recover given a little convalescing time. Those who develop no feelings of nausea, however, and instead discover blood in their underwear in the next seventy-two hours, will have no such luck. These unfortunate victims will have contracted the full-blown disease, will have no natural immunity whatsoever and should prepare to die in a most hideous, drawn-out fashion at some point over the next two weeks.

It's obvious that two things would happen after this announcement. The first is that people would become convinced they were about to see blood and would find themselves in a state of hyperventilation every time they went for a pee, mustering every last ounce of mental stamina to peer into the toilet bowl or to stand under fluorescent lighting scrutinising their used toilet paper, cursing their partners for the red polka-dotted roll of tissue they so stupidly bought on sale from the local supermarket.

'Does this look like blood to you?' people would ask desperately, holding out urine-soaked squares of toilet paper for their friends and families to inspect.

The second thing to happen would be everyone hoping and praying that they were about to feel violently sick. And if you think about feeling queasy for long enough, it's safe to say that eventually you'll start to experience it. Even if your brain won't agree to psychosomatically induce an episode of hurling, the knowledge of the fate lying in store for you if you don't start to demonstrate a positive symptom pretty damned soon would be enough to make most people lose their last meal.

Of course, the great advantage to the global red-alert state of biological warfare scenario is that everyone on the planet would be descending into this sort of madness together. Whereas when you're stuck in the IVF two-week wait, you, and you alone, are the raving nutjob.

7.30pm

This afternoon, Nat and I wandered into town again on a short shopping expedition. The purpose of our trip was to buy Valentine's cards for our other halves ahead of next Tuesday – although, I have to confess I kind of struggled to find a card whose tone would befit both the happiest and most miserable day of our lives to date.

A little later, violating my pure, organic diet, we decided to plump for an incredibly unhealthy lunch of pecan and maple syrup waffles in an upmarket, solely dessert-focused restaurant over the road.

The waffles were good. In fact, as the first non-healthy lunch I've eaten in a long time, they were better than good; they were virtually orgasmic.

The ambience, however, was not.

I could swear that at each of the twelve tables in the restaurant, every single customer was either nursing a small baby or resting her hands on her enormous pregnancy bump. Everywhere I turned, big pregnant bellies were rising up out of seats, babies were screaming and prams were being rocked backwards and forwards in the narrow aisles between each table. At one point, amidst the screams of babies and toddlers all around us, I was sure I could even make out the gush of waters breaking against the terracotta floor tiles in the back room.

Looking around, I had to pinch the back of my hand to convince myself that I hadn't developed narcolepsy and fallen into a nightmare, or died without noticing and slipped straight down into hell.

I don't belong here, I told myself with absolute certainty.

It didn't for one second occur to me that I might, in fact, belong here after all, that I might be in the very secret beginning stage of pregnancy, just waiting to bloom like all the glowing pregnant goddesses around me.

In that moment I just knew I was an imposter, like a little girl who's allowed to dress up, draw on red lipstick and traipse around in oversized high heels, but only until her bedtime when she'll be ordered upstairs and all the big girls will go out to the party without her.

In an attempt to suppress the inner turmoil when we arrived back home, I immediately lit a couple of candles, dimmed the lights and inflicted my IVF relaxation CD upon Nat, so she too could have the pleasure of being instructed to visualise Kenneth and Donaghy burrowing into my welcoming womb.

That bloody CD worked a treat for Nat, and within seconds she'd slipped into a blissful, pregnancy-induced snooze, snoring softly in time to the whale song, her body eager, I imagine, to snatch any opportunity to reverse the ruining effects of motherhood.

The whale song, unsurprisingly, worked no such magic upon me.

So after thirty minutes I gave up, got up and made a start on dinner. And when Nat woke up we took our pregnancy vitamins together just like before and, again, I wondered what the hell I was doing and why on earth I was going through the motions of doing all these things that are so very unnecessary for someone in my clearly un-pregnant state.

I mean, this is fucking pathetic, isn't it? I may as well be walking around with a prosthetic pregnancy bump strapped to my stomach or a cushion shoved up my jumper.

I'm so disappointed in myself that I'm not managing to enjoy the experience of being potentially pregnant more than I am. Every time we've been through IVF I've felt determined to get some enjoyment from this possibly pregnant state and from the knowledge that we are so tantalisingly close.

But once I'm back here again in the thick of it, I know there's no hope of ever enjoying this situation. The reality is that I'm no longer a little kid; I'm a grown, thirty-five-year-old woman, and there can be no fulfilment or fun anymore to be found in dressing up.

11.50pm

Something truly terrible has happened.

Well, allow me to elaborate: something has happened which has truly terrible repercussions for me; for everyone else I imagine it's just fucking peachy.

Well, that's not really true; in reality, it has no repercussions for me whatsoever.

No? So why then does it feel as though a bomb has just exploded in my face?

Okay…deep breaths now…

In the communal hallway of our flats this evening, DH had a brief conversation with our neighbours, Doug and Alex, the upshot of which is that they are expecting their first baby in just under three months' time.

This news, as DH delivered it second-hand, hit me like a sledgehammer between the eyes, and it was a few seconds before I could even draw breath to speak.

I swallowed. 'Well, that explains why she's been looking so fat, then,' I spat eventually.

It also explained quite a few other things, like why Doug had been making so much noise all afternoon as he carted boxes of furniture in and out through their front door.

I'd half wondered at the time if they were splitting up and one of them was moving out…but no, that would be too much to hope for, wouldn't it?

No, they weren't splitting up and squabbling over the material spoils of their shattered relationship like any nice, self-respecting couple. Instead, they'd been sneaking around behind our backs all this time, slyly getting pregnant and then clearing out their spare room so they could build a fucking nursery in its place.

I stared at the wall of our living room, behind which I knew the traitorous bastards would be hiding.

'YOU SELFISH MOTHERFUCKERS!' I suddenly shouted at the top of my voice.

All this time we've been thinking that the stork hadn't heard of our postal code and wouldn't deliver this side of the river, and then tonight we find out that he does deliver to our very doorstep, but that some other fucker just pilfered our package before we got home one day.

'Did you manage to say something conventional?' I asked DH, feeling my face flush a brilliant red as the blood visibly frothed beneath the surface of my skin.

'Of course I did,' he replied, eyeing me disapprovingly, 'I'm not you, remember.'

'I'm not me either,' I snapped at him. 'Not really. Well, not in public anyway.'

Although I'm worried I might have been the real me – and in public – had I heard this glorious news first-hand this evening.

'Oh, you have to be FUCKING kidding me!' I might have screamed before shaking my head, tutting and stomping off into the flat.

I can't believe I'd been toying with the idea of inviting Doug and Alex round for a long-overdue get-to-know-you drink a few weeks ago. But after some contemplation I'd eventually decided against the idea, concluding that I'd rather appear standoffish or antisocial than invite them over for a mulled wine and then have to slink off into the kitchen to grab my nightly injection from the fridge while no one was looking. Or have to decline a mulled wine myself, without providing any plausible reason for not drinking one, and risk being asked if I was pregnant.

Imagine if I'd decided to go ahead with the invitation: they'd have arrived at the door and, too late, I'd have been confronted by the great enormous bump. And then in she'd have waddled, plonking herself down on our sofa and guzzling all of our orange juice while I grinned at her maniacally and asked her thoughtful and interested questions about her impending delivery of undiluted fucking joy.

Jesus, two minutes in and I'd have wanted to smash a bottle of mulled wine over both their heads and bury the smug bastards in our communal backyard.

Standing beside the paper-thin wall that conjoins our living rooms, I screamed as loudly as possible about how I hoped Doug and Alex are urgently looking for somewhere else to live. Because if they're not then we're going to have to find somewhere else to live ourselves…which is just fucking fantastic because I really liked this fucking flat and I don't want to fucking start searching for somewhere new, and we'd never fucking well be accepted as tenants now anyway because neither of us has a fucking steady job, and besides we need to save every last fucking penny we can scrape together for our next fucking round of IVF treatment. But I guess we'll fucking have to move out if these fuckers are planning to stay put. Which they obviously fucking are, because I've just fucking watched them cart the entire fucking contents of a brand-new fucking nursery through their fucking front door.

How can they do this to us?

'HOW CAN YOU DO THIS TO US?' I want to yell at them through the wall.

I've not been able to stop myself from working through the calculations in my head. If they are due in May, then they must have conceived in August – the month that we underwent our second ill-fated cycle of IVF.

At the end of that punishing month I stood alone in our bathroom, tearfully searching through the cabinet for yet another packet of sanitary towels that I'd hoped I wouldn't need, while just feet away, unbeknownst to me, another couple must have been excitedly jumping up and down at the sight of their positive pregnancy test.

I wouldn't have believed before tonight that it was possible to feel so betrayed by people whose first names I barely know and who've done absolutely nothing except innocently get on with living their own lives.

But what's truly unbelievable in all of this is that the news has just struck me like a bolt from the blue tonight. I've developed something of a dark talent over the years for predicting when these announcements are due. I've pencilled them all into a schedule I hold in my head, so I can prepare for whoever's first, second or third announcement is likely to be coming up next.

But this one wasn't on my radar. And my ignorance of it only makes me feel even more of a fool and a failure than I normally do, even though, in reality, it makes no difference whatsoever whether or not I get to scream 'I fucking knew it!' when this kind of news is broken to me.

Tonight's revelation only confirms something that I have long suspected: that this world is turning into one giant conspiracy against me.

And although it involves two people who mean virtually nothing to us, people we know only to nod to outside the door of our flat and exchange pleasantries with some mornings, this is strangely one of the most hurtful pregnancy announcements of all.

I can see, suddenly, the next few months unfolding before me in an eerie kind of slow motion, like a car crash that I'm powerless to prevent.

We'll watch from the window as Doug and Alex arrive home from hospital with their carefully wrapped bundle, we'll see pink or blue balloons appear on their front door, we'll witness the processions of family and friends turning up to welcome the new arrival, and I'll bump into her at the bottom of the stairwell every single sodding day, right before she skips away on a carefree jaunt through the town with her gorgeous new pram, and I trudge off to my 368th fertility consultation.

And then at night, I will lie awake listening to Doug and Alex's baby stirring and crying, almost as though it is lying in a Moses basket in our very own room. *Almost.*

And this baby's nightly cries will eventually form the backing track to the dread and the fear that pound through my heart as I lie in bed waiting for the menopause to come and claim me, while hopelessly trying to convince myself that I don't need to experience motherhood to feel complete.

1.05am

Two cups of decaffeinated tea and a whole lot of crap TV later and I still feel enraged enough to power the country's energy supply through my blood pressure alone.

Whether or not they're expected, these announcements don't get any easier. I know deep down that it's just something amazing and exciting that's happening to another couple – or even in some cases, something that's deemed neither amazing nor exciting, but something that's happening to the ungrateful wankers nonetheless.

It doesn't change the fact, though, that it feels like some kind of malevolent cosmic joke that's being played on us. When these announcements first hit, I can't put into words the feelings that rise up and threaten to overwhelm me.

Well, *I* could have a pretty good crack at putting it into words actually, if anyone was interested to know.

It feels as though someone has reached into my body, ripped out my womb and stolen all our future babies with it. It no longer feels as though people are telling me they're having *their* baby; it feels as though they're telling me they're having *mine.* They're having one *instead* of us having one. We've waited years in a queue, patiently holding out for our turn, and every time we get to the front, a whole truckload of fuckers, some of whom would claim to be our family and friends, barge in front and elbow us right to the back again. Some of them have enjoyed their 'turn' once, twice, even three times on the trot now; why can't they let us have just one lousy go?

DH will tell me, as he has for the hundredth time tonight, that I mustn't let these announcements get under my skin. But he does not understand.

He can't know how it feels to be pouring blood, sweat, tears and money we don't have into trying to achieve a positive pregnancy test, while women all around me are doing it with their eyes closed, nonchalantly ticking it off their to-do list before breakfast, sometimes even unconsciously doing it by mistake.

Well, admittedly he has *some* idea of all of this, of course. And I can see a shadow of the blackness I'm feeling etched on his face tonight; that kind of winded, shocked expression you wear when you've just unexpectedly walked into a door.

He would never, ever admit to it, though.

Before tonight, I actually felt reassured that I was getting better at handling other people's jubilant declarations, that my bilious alter-ego was growing a little subdued in her old age. But now I realise that I just haven't been tested by a jubilant declaration for a while – and that my bilious alter-ego is very much alive and is in fact wound like a tightly coiled spring, ready to spew out a lifetime's supply of turbo-strength venom in the face of the next happily expectant mother she encounters.

I know I have nothing left to say to people like Doug and Alex; the well from which I've been fishing for the appropriate and conventional remarks has officially run dry.

So next time someone whispers to me, all tentative, eyes glistening, 'We've just found out we're pregnant…again!' all that will be left in my arsenal will be to sigh, shake my head and tell them, 'Well, fuck you too, then.'

At the next christening or blessing I attend I could well find myself leaping up out of my seat and bombing down the aisle with my own A Capella rendition of 'IT SHOULD'VE BEEN ME!'

I won't be held responsible if something like this happens from now on. I simply can't do this anymore.

2.00am

A quick appraisal of my behaviour over the course of tonight makes it clear to me that I need a baby to come into my life very soon. I can't go on like this.

I know of course that I *won't* go on like this. This hateful alter-ego who's surfacing from within must be tied down with rocks and drowned somewhere in the depths of my soul. She's far too ugly to unleash in public. And she's far too ugly to unleash in private, too. DH has told me on many occasions now that he has no desire to see her – and neither, for that matter, do I.

But her strength scares me on nights like tonight. Because I hear her rattling her chains, feel her rising up, and I'm not sure I can stop her if she decides she's breaking free.

3.00am

I'm still wide awake. Well, how can I sleep after tonight's events?

Thank God Nat had already gone to bed before DH shared his unwelcome newsflash with me. Although she would have needed to be in a pregnancy-induced coma to have missed all the shouting and screaming that ensued.

I can't imagine what I'll say if she asks about it in the morning. I mean, I can't inform a pregnant person that this is simply how I respond to pregnancy announcements, can I?

I hope to God that DH is going to be around to drive Nat back to the coach station tomorrow morning. If the traffic's bad, it could easily take an hour and a half in the car and, on top of being drunk on a sour cocktail of bitterness, frustration and rage, aimed largely at our next door neighbours, I'm now severely sleep-deprived to boot.

I am not up to the job of driving a car. And I'm most definitely not up to the job of driving a car containing a heavily pregnant woman.

Killing myself in a head-on collision is one thing. I can live with that.

But killing my pregnant friend is quite another.

I mean, aside from the obvious tragedy, what the hell would people think?

Day Eleven — Friday 10th February

Scraping the Bottom of the Tea Leaves

Symptoms: Very sore boobs (pessary-related, I am certain), constipation, extreme tiredness, and a barely controllable compulsion to order our neighbours into a removal van and insist that they vacate their property at once!

Remaining hours: 96 (We're under the 100 mark at last and on the home stretch now. But on the home stretch to which destination? That is the question.)

Waking hours remaining: 64

Predicted odds on this working: 1/10

6.45am

Well, that was awkward.

It's bin collection day today and, as luck would have it, just as I stepped outside to wheel our bin down to the end of our front garden, who should be standing there in her dressing gown but Alex. A very obviously pregnant Alex, I should add.

So, it's true then, I thought to myself, furiously. And then I wondered why Doug wasn't wheeling out the bin and leaving his very pregnant girlfriend to relax in bed.

And *then* I remembered what Alex had done to me and that she should by rights be in chains right now, emptying dog litter bins with her teeth.

'Morning!' I yelled at her with almost hysterical-sounding false cheer.

Alex gave me a tired, pregnant smile in response and made to shuffle back into her house, holding her aching back in that infuriating way that pregnant women do, like they expect somebody to award them a rosette each time they manage to leave their chair.

Not so fast, I thought as she tottered up the steps to our shared front door. She had some serious explaining to do and I wanted to know exactly what she had to say for herself. And yes, I was perfectly prepared to stand outside in -1°C conditions in my dressing gown freezing my nipples off in order to hear it.

'Not long to go now, then!' I shouted, nodding towards her bulging belly.

How had I not noticed that enormous barrel beneath her jumper before? It's true I hadn't seen her in a while, but come on! I mean, I've started to notice (and feel pangs of jealously towards) pregnant squirrels in the last couple of years. This just doesn't make sense.

'Yeah, not long enough,' she replied, smiling but looking down anxiously at her bump as she spoke.

'Not long enough for *what*?' I hissed, sensing that a vein in my forehead had suddenly started to pulse.

'Oh, you know,' she continued, running a hand through her unbrushed hair to emphasise her pregnancy-induced unkemptness, 'there's just so much still to do and we're really not prepared. To be honest I just didn't think we'd be having a baby in this flat, so, you know, it's just come as a bit of a surprise.'

'Wow,' I said to her, 'why don't you wait here for a second while I go and find a large stick for you? Then I'll come back and hand it over so you can jab it repeatedly into my eye socket for the next ten minutes – because, you know what? That would actually be a lot less painful than standing here and listening to one more syllable of this CONVERSATION!'

Okay, so that's not exactly what I said – well, not out loud, anyway.

I think what I actually opted for in response was something to the effect of, 'Oh, I'm sure it will all come together just fine. It always does when you've got a deadline, doesn't it?'

Yeah, like I'd know anything about meeting baby-making deadlines!

'What's the matter with you?' DH asked as I slammed the front door and stormed back into the flat.

'They're having our baby,' I told him, pointing through the living-room wall to where Alex and Doug, the baby snatchers, were lurking.

'What?'

'They are. She just told me. She just admitted it to my face. She said they didn't even order one, and they were surprised to find out they were getting one in May. There's obviously been a mix-up. We ordered one; it got delivered next door instead. Probably happens a lot.'

'Oh, God,' DH groaned, rolling his eyes skyward.

'I'm simply reporting a serious incidence of unintentional theft involving our next-door neighbours,' I told him.

'Oh, great, the crazy woman has returned,' DH yelled before he grabbed his jacket and informed me he was heading out to the gym. 'Please get rid of this crazy, hysterical woman and bring my wife back by the time I get home,' he roared over his shoulder.

As he left he slammed the door behind him with such force that the windows at the front of the flat rattled loudly in their frames.

'Morning!' I heard him bellow with startling merriment in the very next breath, obviously passing Doug in the hallway on his way to work.

Christ, our neighbours must think we're complete and utter sociopaths.

And just then, I became aware of someone standing behind me in the living room.

'Is it okay if I get a bowl of porridge?' Nat murmured, nervously poking her head round the door.

Oh, yes. Other people. I must remember other people, mustn't I? Must try to keep the crazy, rabid, frothing-at-the-mouth version of myself nailed down to something solid while other people are in the vicinity. Especially pregnant people. They are particularly vulnerable, aren't they?

4.00pm

Luckily, since DH has been asked to work this Saturday, he's been given today off in lieu, which meant he was available to drive Nat and me to the coach station this morning.

And I'm relieved to report that there were no instances of cars being wrapped around trees or other inopportune accidents.

In fact, the middle section of our journey was both surprisingly and spectacularly beautiful, the sky lit by a brilliant low-hanging sun that cast dazzling rays across the streets, trees and rows of hedges that had been meticulously frosted in white.

No matter which way I looked, I couldn't help but wonder whether we had been somehow transported from our south London suburb to the magical land of Narnia.

And yet even this could not override the realisation that I am falling apart at the seams.

I wish I knew what to do to make this awful feeling go away. But I fear that a positive pregnancy test might be the only known cure.

Before she left to catch her coach back home, Nat hugged DH and me tightly and wished us luck for next week, telling us she's still holding out hope that our pregnancies will overlap, if only now for a few short months.

It's been good to see her at this terrible time, even though she was powerless to stop the last few days from being a truly terrible time.

I know that Nat wants this interminably depressing chapter in my life to come to an end almost as much as I do. She wants to return to simply being friends again, without having to tiptoe around this immense pile of awkwardness and guilt and resentment that lies between us.

But waiting and hoping for this interminably depressing chapter to be over isn't what's important anymore. What matters is that we've spent these last few days together *in spite of it all,* and in doing so we've acknowledged and agreed that we are just going to grit our teeth and get through this somehow.

It seems we've mutually and wordlessly accepted that the time we spend together doesn't need to be like the good old times and it doesn't even need to be fun; sometimes it's enough to simply say that we did our duty and got it done.

It was so kind of Nat to say that she still believes things will work out for us and we'll have our family soon.

Many people have casually assured me over the years that it will definitely all work out in the end, but far fewer would say it now; it's really just the hardcore believers like DH, my mother, Jen, Nat and a couple of other close friends, but I'll never grow tired of the people I love telling me about their firm beliefs and positive feelings.

I mean, it goes without saying that they're the lousiest psychics on earth, with a track record of false predictions that does little to inspire confidence. But their unwavering belief in the happy ending that's waiting just around the corner is still the greatest kindness that anyone has shown to me throughout this five-year trial.

I've combed the country's fertility clinics for a doctor who might show even half this level of encouragement, but nobody so far has obliged. Peddling false hope is a trick that only a doctor of the lowest moral integrity would employ, and so they prefer to honestly confront us with bleak statistical diagrams that demonstrate how, with a set protocol, situations have sometimes turned around for other couples whose problems might not be completely different from our own.

I remember a couple of years ago, having failed to unearth the fertility specialist who'd tell me what I wanted to hear, I resorted to visiting a *proper* psychic, someone who might, for a small fee, be happier to indulge me in the prognosis I wanted to be given.

And so one Tuesday afternoon I did the previously unthinkable and caught the Tube into Central London for an appointment with my carefully selected tarot card reader.

I can still remember the rational fragment of my brain berating me at each and every stop along the way for doing something so desperate – but still I did not turn back.

Christina the tarot card reader was surprisingly down to earth, as it turned out. She fit the stereotypical image in terms of her long black hair, tie-dyed skirt and purple velvet waistcoat, but in many ways the experience felt similar to chatting to a friend over a casual cup of coffee.

The only difference was that we were sitting in a small basement under a dusty bookstore, a few joss sticks burning in the background to help muster a general ambience of mysticism.

'So, you desperately want a baby,' she told me within seconds of uncovering my first card.

I nodded, mutely.

'Well, that's not happening at the moment,' she continued, in such a decisive tone that I had to glance beneath the table to check that she hadn't slipped a celestial internal probe inside my vagina to assess the contents of my uterus without my noticing.

She went on to tell me, rather gravely, that I needed to inject more fun into my life or my marriage would soon start to crumble. And her warning was immediately followed by the suggestion that DH and I take up tantric sex lessons (run by her saggy-bollocked co-worker Sensual Seth, I imagined) to help keep our staid old love life fresh and interesting.

Oh, I can't wait to suggest this to DH, I smiled inwardly, whilst trying my hardest to look as though I was giving the idea some serious consideration.

'Well, things haven't been *too* bad in that department,' I tried to reassure her, weakly, keen to quickly brush this awkward topic aside.

'Hmmm, I think they have,' she insisted, 'I think they've been very bad indeed.'

Holy crap! Here I was sitting across a coffee table from this woman and she was apparently 'seeing' my sex life being played out before her eyes. And if that was true then I knew in that instant that her vision must have transported her to that regrettable incident months earlier involving the five gallons of sperm-friendly lubricant.

I was sorely tempted to point out that there were definitely better examples than that one, and that if she would only select a different sex tape from our back catalogue then she would surely agree that things weren't always so dire.

But I was keen to move away from a further dissection of my love life, so I confided in her that I was worried we were never going to become parents, frantically hoping that she would retract her statement from a few moments before about it 'not happening', and instead smile at me knowingly and urge me to pick up a pregnancy test on my way home that night.

But rather than saying anything along those lines, she just stopped dead and asked me, 'Well, what do *you* think will happen? How would *you* answer the question if you asked yourself whether you were ever going to be a mother?'

Right on cue, I burst into tears – probably a useful response in hindsight, since my gulping and snivelling pretty much rendered me mute for the remainder of her reading.

'Look, you're a highly intuitive person,' she added, wafting a couple of tissues in my direction, 'and I know you know the answer to this question if you look inside your heart.'

But I only shook my head in response, because I didn't, and I don't, know what my heart feels anymore.

'How old are you anyway?' she asked me, once I had finally regained some composure. 'Thirty-seven, thirty-eight, right?'

'Thirty-*three*!' I wailed and made another grab for the tissues.

I was starting to wonder by this point why exactly I was paying this stranger to insult me and make me cry, when I had an office full of people back at work who would have happily done it for free – and without my even needing to ask.

'Thirty-three?' she continued. 'You're so *young*! You've got nothing to worry about. Christ, think how I feel. I'm *forty*-three and I'm still wondering if I'm ever going to have a baby.'

Well, you're the fucking fortune teller, I wanted to remind her; can't you just turn over a few cards or something? Or take yourself next door for a healing tantric sex lesson with Sensual Seth?

Since this (my first and only) appointment with a crystal ball, I've been forced to concede that I will not find one person on this planet who will be able to tell me, with any degree of authority, that everything is going to be okay.

And so I have had to accept that, as much as I cannot bear it for a single second longer, I must somehow learn to live alongside this uncertainty.

9.00pm

Okay, I'll admit it: I'm starting to cringe a little when I look back at how I reacted to Doug and Alex's news last night, and again this morning on the driveway.

Don't get me wrong, I'm nowhere near as ashamed of myself as I ought to be, but a small part of me has been left shaking her head disapprovingly at the way I've handled this situation.

Things need to change. *I* need to change. I need to reaffirm all those promises that DH and I made when we escaped to the coast for a few days after our second failed IVF cycle.

During the course of several ten-kilometre uphill walks – walks that our bodies barely registered because we had so many brain-engulfing cobwebs that needed to be blown away – we agreed that we absolutely *must* start participating in our lives again. We had to pursue other interests, find fun wherever it was hiding and accept that our lives were just going to be different from how we'd imagined.

Achieving this peaceful state of mind is a goal I've been pursuing ever since, but most of the time it seems as though the closer it appears one day, the further away it slips the next.

I now realise, if I'm ever to make my peace with never holding our baby in my arms, there are many other hurtful truths that I must come to terms with first.

I must accept the reality that the friends, family members and acquaintances all around us will continue to get pregnant and to extend their family units. Those who already have one or two babies will go on to have three or four, and those who currently have none will all make the grand leap into parenthood and establish their new lives with children.

It's quite possible that *all* of the duplicitous fuckers will do it: the friends who've yet to meet the mother or father of their future children, the family members who are still in their late teens and not even thinking about having kids yet, the bachelors and spinsters everyone assumed would stay single forever, and even the people we know who genuinely don't want children in their lives but will end up being coerced or duped into parenthood by a persuasive or devious partner.

Like tidal waves, these announcements, births and transitions will slam into us one by one, and it's now a personal challenge for me to find a way to let them wash straight over my head, to withstand them like a rock face, never allowing them to knock me off my feet.

I must also make my peace with the fact that I may never be able to participate in those conversations women love to have about pregnancy, childbirth and motherhood.

And I must find a way to visit friends and family and share in the celebrations of their new arrivals, content in the knowledge that while I'll never be able to experience the joy first-hand, I can still feel warmed by my involvement in other people's happy times.

I must learn to fearlessly anticipate questions from friends, family, acquaintances and total strangers about our ~~childless~~ child-free state, and respond with a calm and disciplined honesty that is not intended to provoke guilt or pity or general social discomfort.

I must accept the unavoidable fact that DH and I will continue to grow older. And that with every passing month and year, my ovaries will wither, my fertility will plummet and our chances of a miracle natural conception will become ever more remote.

I must learn to stop hyperventilating in the face of this ageing process, to forgive my defective body for stubbornly withholding the gift that DH and I felt so certain it held in store. I must learn to grow old and ever more infertile with dignity and with grace.

Lastly, and possibly hardest of all, I must accept the certainty that new investigations and treatments will continue to become available, and I will never know whether this one or that one or a collaboration of them all would have provided the answer to this riddle that has tortured me for so long.

When these discoveries and breakthroughs emerge and bring relief to other couples (future versions of us), I must resist the urge to wonder whether it's too late to give it one last shot, and whether with the highest dose of fertility drugs known to man, we might still be able to dredge up one last egg with which to conceive our long-awaited baby.

Instead, I must smile, shrug and feel satisfied in my heart that having a baby just wasn't in my life plan, that our greyhound's development would be disrupted by a new family member now anyway, and that things are perfectly okay as they stand.

11.50pm

Lying in bed tonight, I've found myself remembering and replaying something that Nat said to me during her stay.

She turned to me yesterday, as we were walking back from lunch, and told me, 'You know, you really couldn't do any more than you're doing to make this happen.'

She added that I'd done so much more than she or anyone she knew had done, or probably would ever do, to get pregnant and that if it still didn't work now, at least I'd know there was nothing else I could possibly have tried.

Aside from telling me that I'll absolutely one hundred per cent get pregnant one day, her words were probably the most comforting thing that anyone has said to me over the last five years.

They are the antithesis of all those awful suggestions and insinuations that if only I were less stressed, could forget about it all, took this or that pill, tried this or that theory or generally practised more good deeds for my fellow man, then perhaps some remunerating god might bestow upon me a suitable reward.

Rather than imply that I must have overlooked or bungled some important step along the way, I think Nat may be the only person to stand shoulder to shoulder with me, to look my failures in the eye and to shake her head in disbelief and contempt; to insist that by rights it absolutely has to work out this time.

Day Twelve — Saturday 11th February
Back to Earth with a Bump (or is That without a Bump?)

Symptoms: A vaguely sore throat. I think I might be coming down with something.
Hours remaining: 72
Waking hours remaining: 48
Predicted odds on this working: 3/10

7.00am

Even though it was still pitch black outside, I found myself wide awake at 6.00am and bursting for a wee, so I hopped quietly out of bed, pulled on my woolly slippers and crept next door to the bathroom.

Before I had time to question what I was about to do, I tiptoed over to the cabinet, pulled out a pregnancy test (which was strange as I could have sworn I'd hidden them under the chest of drawers in our spare room at the start of this two-week wait), ripped open the packet and peed in the plastic measuring jug that I keep by the side of the toilet for such occasions (not one that I'd ever interchange with the kitchen measuring jug, I hasten to add; this one's uses are strictly confined to HCG detection).

Balancing the measuring jug on my knee, I promptly dipped the test stick into the liquid and held it there while I slowly counted to ten.

When the ten seconds were up, instead of turning the test face down and fleeing the bathroom like I normally would, sneaking back minutes later to try to flip it over from the furthest possible distance – kind of like a desperately hungry lion attempting to maul a highly venomous snake – I just held it centimetres from my face, and watched, unblinking, as the urine swam through the clear rectangular window in a pink haze and settled into a single concentrated line to the right-hand side of the stick.

I continued to stare at it, unflinching, passive, ambivalent almost, not willing it to do anything in particular, just watching with interest to see what would happen next.

And as I watched, a pale pink line began to emerge to the left of the other, faint as a watercolour at first, and then growing stronger and stronger, like a face rising up out of a lake to greet me. When the picture finally settled, I was left gazing at a small plastic stick with two distinct lines, just like the ones they show in adverts, the ones that other women hold in their hands every single day.

So, this was it, then: the sight for sore eyes, the pot of gold at the end of the rainbow, the moment for which I'd been holding my breath for five long years.

I started to laugh out loud and then to cry and scream and laugh again, until DH came blundering in, disorientated and terrified, a look on his face that suggested he was expecting to find either a burglar or some kind of monstrous insect in the bathroom with me.

'I got my BFP, I got my BFP!' I cried.

Even as the words were leaving my mouth, I couldn't help thinking that they were an odd choice; I couldn't recall ever having used the expression 'BFP' with anyone other than my Tarantino buddies.

'I knew it, I just *knew* it!' I continued to cry as he picked me up and spun me around the bathroom.

Had I known it? I sure as hell didn't remember 'knowing it' over the last few days; in fact if anything I remember feeling distinctly pessimistic about our chances of a happy outcome.

But who cared, right? All that had gone before was suddenly irrelevant; I just needed to focus on this one awe-inspiring, incredible moment.

And then, before I quite knew what was happening, we were in my parents' living room and I was screaming to them that I had my BFP, which again seemed peculiar as I'm certain neither one of them would have ever encountered the expression in their lives – not to mention the unwelcome fact that my dad had died two years earlier.

But somehow he was sat there in his old, familiar armchair, alive and well, and they both instantly understood what I was talking about, and within seconds of hearing the news they were bringing out all the gifts they'd been storing in the cupboard under their stairs over the last few years and piling them up in a big tower in front of us. It was a Jenga-style monument of carry cots, highchairs, baby clothes and toys.

I fought with all my might to focus on the presents in front of us, but I couldn't seem to stop them from sliding in and out of focus, and my attention was frustratingly being drawn elsewhere, towards the sound of an alarm, somewhere to my right, and also what could only be a newsreader's voice, talking reproachfully about the many failings within the adoption system in the UK.

In the instant my eyes opened, my heart sank like a stone. So, my dad isn't…no, don't be stupid. And I'm not actually…no. Well, no, of course not.

But somehow, in amongst the confusion and disappointment, as I peeled my head off the pillow and saw DH slurping back a mouthful of coffee as he hurriedly dressed for work, I found an unexpected yet unmistakable sense of hope surging forward from deep within.

I couldn't recall ever having experienced a dream like this one before. It felt as though my body was sending me a message, telling me that this time it had done what it was supposed to do. And in that moment I just knew. And it was completely different to all the times I had 'just known' in the past.

'Wait there,' I whispered to DH, as I clambered out of bed and rushed past him to the bathroom.

Just as in the dream, I pulled out a test from the top shelf of the bathroom cabinet (damn it, I really *had* left them in there all along), peed into the measuring jug, held the test stick in the liquid for a good ten seconds, and then placed it down on the edge of the bathtub.

And then without even waiting for the result, I picked up the stick and carried it through to DH, who had stopped getting ready for work and was standing very still, just staring at the TV.

'I got my BFP,' I whispered, as I went to stand beside him, taking his hand in mine. And then I looked down at the stick and saw two strong pink lines staring back at me. It was the exact image I had seen in my dream world just moments before.

My God, I thought, I must have felt confident to give DH that piece of news before I'd even looked at the result.

'I know,' DH said, squeezing my hand tightly but continuing to stare vacantly at the TV screen ahead.

And then the next thing I knew I was back in the bathroom, kneeling down on the floor beside the toilet with my phone in my hand, this time screaming to Nat, 'I got my BFP, I got my BFP!'

And it was at that precise point that the front door slammed downstairs and I jolted awake to find the alarm ringing in my ear and the TV blaring out an interview about the adoption crisis in the UK.

Fuck. Of course it had been too good to be true.

It *did* account for all my unusual behaviour, though: shouting my head off about BFPs and revealing test results before they had even been confirmed.

Damn it. Damn it. DAMN IT! The best thing that's happened to me in recent memory – possibly ever – and it turns out to be nothing more than a fucking fantasy.

Obviously, there was no question that I was properly awake after that. You may not always know for sure when you are dreaming, but you sure as shit know when you're back in the real world.

Dreams wrapped up in dreams, sometimes wrapped up in yet more dreams, are not uncommon for me around the time I'm supposed to be getting up, and I remember that they became a regular occurrence back when I was commuting to work in the City.

Before today, though, they've always revolved around mundane activities, like getting up, getting dressed and travelling halfway across London. That kind of self-deception used to be maddening enough, when in reality my alarm had gone off an hour earlier and I was still tucked up cosily in bed and lying face down in a puddle of my own contented drool. But it was nowhere near as devastating as finally getting to celebrate the pregnancy we've waited for all these years – *and* with a parent I thought I'd never get to tell – only to discover that I actually still have another two days to wait before finding out that we are probably not pregnant yet again.

This time my twisted subconscious has truly surpassed itself.

11.30am

It seems the inevitable 'toilet terror' which accompanies every IVF two-week wait has begun in earnest today.

My period is due in two days' time, but I know that if the pessaries don't keep it at bay, and there's nothing exciting like a pregnancy to stop it in its tracks, then those first telltale spots of blood could be making an appearance any time from now.

Each time I venture to the bathroom for a pee, I have to counsel myself to stand up, wipe and whip the toilet paper up plainly in front of my eyes to confront any tinges of colour that may be present.

I wonder how many more toilet trips I will need to make before our official test date. Far too many for comfort, I know that for certain.

I've found myself talking to Kenneth and Donaghy a lot today, asking them to send me a signal that they're still alive, that they're managing to hang on in there somehow.

What's causing my distinctly not-pregnant feelings, I'd like to know. Is it an instinctive acknowledgement that it really is time to start grieving the loss of our genetic children? Or are these feelings only a manifestation of my very worst fears?

I keep reminding myself that fear is a powerful emotion and that it's only human nature to dread the disappearance of the people and the things that we want and need the most.

But what I'm sensing in the pit of my stomach, the nothingness that is permeating my body from the womb outwards, feels both distressingly real and heart-sinkingly familiar.

I fear it is more than just the fear that is talking to me now.

12.30pm

I received a text message a little while ago from an old workmate, a girl called Molly whom I met when we both worked Saturdays in a small art shop near Notting Hill. She apologised for the short notice, but asked me if I'd like to help her celebrate her birthday tonight, at a cocktail bar not far from here.

She already knows I will decline, because history dictates I always will, but I am more grateful to her than she could ever imagine for continuing to send these invites nevertheless.

Truth be told, I would love nothing more than a cocktail with

Molly tonight; a chance to get warm and fuzzy with this happy-go-lucky, good-time party girl; to block out all the worry and the pain; to show my dear friend of fifteen years, in actions not just words, how much I value her loveliness and her loyalty and her determination to keep me in her life.

But it is not a good time.

It is NEVER a good time anymore.

I couldn't begin to explain this to Molly, but today I have been forced to accept that I am now locked in a private and solitary hell until this verdict is given.

There is no way I can be in any other human's company when a simple trip to the toilet could crush my very will to go on living.

There have been other invitations over the last few days: Jen has offered to take me on countless outings, my mum (either guessing what's going on or having already been told by Jen) has offered to come over to keep me company, and there have been other messages and missed calls from good people who could probably provide a welcome distraction at what can only be described as 'this difficult time'.

But as our entire future hangs in the balance, I feel the need to sever all connections, to turn into my own tiny corner of the world and to focus all my energy on simply getting through every remaining day, hour by torturous hour, minute by torturous minute, second by torturous second.

DH will be there to join me at the final destination, of course, but the seemingly endless stretch of time between now and then is mine to navigate as I will.

1.30pm

One more cup of decaffeinated tea: one more tiny piece of comfort to help me through the next seventy-two hours without completely losing my mind.

Followed by another inevitable request from my body to empty my bladder, another heart-stopping moment of terror, and another escape from the clutches of the unwanted show of blood.

But for how much longer can my luck hold out?

I have such a lot of spare time on my hands right now; time to play out the various endings to this story, time to contemplate, and I mean *really* contemplate, what we'll do if we never have a child.

We won't be the first people in the world it will have happened to, and nor will we be the last.

The counsellor I visited after our first failed IVF treatment (a pleasant woman named Susan, with wild auburn hair and a hangdog expression) suggested it was the unnamed fears we harbour that have the power to torment us the most. To combat these fears, she explained, we must find a way to give them a voice, push them out into the open and then confront them head-on.

If Susan was right, then at some point I must summon my fears to burst forth from the closet where they've been barricaded all these years, and I must force myself to take a long hard look at them under a spotlight.

And, maybe, since I clearly have nothing better to do, today is the perfect day for me to lift my head above the parapet.

So here goes:

I fear (and I know DH fears it too) that without our children we'll never quite be enough for one another, and that try as we might to fill the void with banknotes, holidays and greyhounds, there will forever be a gaping hole in our lives where the little people should have been.

DH fears that it will all get too much for me and one of these days I'll completely freak out, have a mid-life crisis and run off with a salsa instructor.

I fear (more realistically, I suspect) that one day DH will weigh it all up and come to the conclusion that, much as he loves me, it wasn't worth the sacrifice; that on balance it might have been preferable to marry a woman he liked maybe a little less but who would have borne him the babies whom he'd come to adore more than anyone or anything on the planet.

I fear that upon reaching the above decision, DH will decide to do something about it. And, equally, I fear that he won't, that he will stay stubbornly stuck to me out of a sense of morality or fidelity until one of us at last has the decency to die.

I fear that our mothers will be robbed of their role as doting grandparents and that our nieces and nephews will be robbed of the cousins who should have been their playmates at family gatherings, their fellow sufferers in compulsory Christmas photos, and the only people who would later share their earliest and probably most treasured memories of childhood.

I fear still being alive when there is nobody left on this earth who means the world to me, and nobody to whom I mean the world.

And, some might say trivially, I feel a fear that chills the very bones of me when I consider what on earth I will be doing on Christmas Day if I find myself still alive at the age of ninety-three.

Okay, so this exercise is not helping me at all.

Perhaps I might feel better if I were to compile a list of all the benefits that I can enjoy if I am destined to remain a ~~childless~~ childfree woman. Benefits such as having an intact perineum and a reasonably functioning bladder. Benefits such as being able to take greater financial risks, be more adventurous, and travel to less developed locations in the world. Benefits such as knowing that DH and I will never find ourselves up on a stage in Menorca dancing to 'Agadoo', or being screamed at by entirely ungrateful teenagers that they hate our guts and they wish they had never been born.

Oh, how rich and fulfilling my life would feel if only I could stand back and appreciate the silver that lines my clouds.

9.30pm

When DH walked through the front door tonight, he found me sitting at the table, laptop in front of me, while a sea of smiling little faces stared back out at me from the pages of an adoption website. Each endearing face was accompanied by a list of important facts and a brief personality summary, much like the Battersea Dogs and Cats Home or an adult dating site.

The difference, in this instance, was that we weren't talking about rehousing an elderly cat or flirting with someone for fifteen minutes over a coffee; we were talking about taking the gamble of a lifetime, a gamble on a tiny person we had never met, a person whom we would nevertheless promise to care for and protect until the day we died.

Of course this is exactly what happens when you conceive a biological child, although, up until this very moment, I have never, ever regarded it in those terms.

It felt both unethical and callous to sit scrolling through these parentless children's profiles, dismissing and rejecting most of them on the grounds of a one paragraph write-up. Although of course there were a couple that I would probably have agreed to adopt right then and there, if only someone had handed me the paperwork.

DH was furious to discover me scouring these websites, accusing me of giving up on Kenneth and Donaghy before the results had even come in.

'There are some *really* sweet kids on there, though,' I started to tell him. 'There's this one little boy with ten-inch thick glasses, curly black hair and gappy teeth…'

'The one who wants to be rehomed with his pet hamster if at all possible?' DH interrupted.

'Yeah, that's the one,' I told him. 'He looks a lot like I did before I started wearing contacts and got some braces. I thought I might be able to help him. And you know I've always considered myself a fairly experienced hamster owner so that wouldn't be a problem.'

There wasn't so much as a twitch of a smile on DH's face, and he looked at me as though he'd caught me red-handed, recklessly cheating on the imaginary family that he felt could so easily be within our grasp.

'Sounds like you looked on the adoption site as well, then?' I pointed out to him.

DH shrugged and admitted he'd had a quick browse, his face still tense and unreadable as he headed into the kitchen.

'It was a few months ago now,' he mumbled over his shoulder. 'There was nothing on TV...'

'Oh,' I said.

It was a shock, no, a *bombshell,* to discover that he too had stared out at this same montage of tiny, hopeful faces.

I'd always felt so sure that I did all the worrying for the both of us, forever racing uphill to peer over the crest and prepare for whichever army we'd be battling next, while DH got on with more pressing matters, compartmentalising and convincing himself that everything was going to be fine.

But it turns out the man deserves credit for a whole lot of premature worrying about our future, after all.

Eventually, he agreed to sit down next to me on the sofa, and confessed that the adoption site had scared the crap out of him, too. Reading about the lengthy approval processes and everything that can and probably will go wrong, it had made him wonder if he and, more importantly, if *I,* would have the strength to undergo more investigations, minor victories, uphill struggles and crushing disappointments.

And even if we had the strength, would we ever measure up as prospective parents? What would we do if it emerged that our adopted children weren't what we wanted after all, and if we weren't even close to what they were going to need?

We both agreed that it just seems so much easier when you become a parent the good old-fashioned way, because you simply get up the duff and *then* start worrying about what the fuck you've done when it's far too late to change your mind. With the adoption process, there's just so much time to think, to worry and to talk yourself out of it. Too much time for DH and I to remind ourselves that our parenting skills have not been road-tested, are mostly hypothetical and are based on nothing more substantial than our ability to keep a couple of goldfish alive for a period of around ten months back in 2010.

If we were to be let loose on a child, how can we say with any degree of certainty how things would turn out?

But if we decide that fostering and adoption just aren't for us, then what are we to do?

Our doctors still can't begin to pin down the source of our fertility problems, so even if we were to try a further ten or twenty cycles of IVF, we've no idea whether it might help us to use a) donor eggs, b) donor sperm, c) a surrogate (and it wouldn't be my mother), or d) all of the above.

And it would be a pretty expensive, not to mention emotionally gruelling, experiment to figure out which of the options from A to D might provide the solution.

And if it turned out to be D, then I think for the sanity of myself, DH, our potential children and all the other people we would have to drag in to assist us, I might just have to take the hint that the universe simply does not want this to happen for us.

Fuck. Three days away from what could be the end of this road and we are still standing here with no contingency, no map for the forward journey, no safety net whatsoever.

I don't think I have ever felt so incredibly small. And, seeing every horrifying emotion that I'm feeling reflected back at me through my husband's eyes tonight, I can honestly say that I have never known two grown people to look so completely and utterly lost.

This is not what I wanted for us.

Back on our wedding day all those many moons ago, this is not what I imagined, even for one second, might be lying around the corner. Just as well we didn't know.

And probably just as well that we also don't know what the next corner holds in store.

Day Thirteen – Sunday 12th February

Never Giving Up?

Symptoms: Scarily vivid dreams (heading more in the direction of vampires, zombies and Mad Hatter's tea parties now rather than positive pregnancy tests, but unsettling to wake from nonetheless). It's unconventional as early pregnancy symptoms go, I'll admit, but I noticed this morning that Goldilocks and Snow White are including this one in their daily lists of symptoms so, what the hell, I've decided I'm having it, too.

Hours remaining: 48

Waking hours remaining: 32

Predicted odds on this working: 2/10

8.45am

It's probably just the anxiety and the tiredness and the overwhelming fear, but I really don't feel well today. I feel as though my brain has finally flipped its lid, clambered up out of my scalp, unravelled and wrapped itself around the outside of my head like a hat. I can't say I'd blame it if it had. It's no fun in there anymore.

They should have IVF farms for women like me to book into at times like these; pretty padded cells with flat-screen TVs and row upon row of feel-good DVDs and relaxation CDs, and beautiful gardens and luxury bathrooms with hot taps that would never heat up to embryo boiling temperatures, and gigantic rocking chairs so that we could legitimately sit and rock ourselves backwards and forwards for hours on end without looking completely crazy in the process.

I have been thinking this morning that I *must* be on the cusp of staging some sort of comeback from this half decade of hibernation and madness. Either I'm going to start attending NCT classes, breastfeeding support groups, baby massage courses and Rhyme Time sessions, and encountering first-hand 'the ten kinds of mothers you meet at playgroups', or I am going to have to find some other reason to drag myself out of bed every morning and to get myself back out into the world.

If only there was something that I was outstandingly good at, or even interested in. Something other than not getting pregnant, that is. That seems to be the one and only area in my thirty-five years on this earth where I've proven to be quite simply fucking phenomenal. And unwaveringly committed.

I wish I had a few other fucking phenomenal skills for my CV. I really could do with discovering a couple quite soon.

10.30am

The mere thought of taking the pregnancy test in two days' time causes my stomach to flip like a giant fish each time it enters my head. This time, I can imagine our official test date coming and going, and those test sticks still lying untouched in their wrappers beneath the chest of drawers in our spare room.

But I know by now that there's no actual risk of that happening. I've yet to encounter a single woman who hasn't taken the test by the time her designated D-day draws to a close. I'd go as far as to bet that it has yet to happen in the thirty-year history of IVF.

In the end, your tormented, frazzled brain can officially take no more, and, for the sake of your very sanity, you are forced to confront the truth, whatever that may be.

DH has nipped to the local shop to grab some unnecessary but hopefully uplifting treats (a newspaper for himself and a chocolate croissant for me), because he knows, from our fourteen years together, that this kind of gesture is the surest way to guarantee at least a fleeting smile on my face. And it was as I was stood by the door, watching him wrap up for the expedition in his hat, scarf and gloves, that, with no warning whatsoever, I suddenly felt that my heart might be about to break.

How has this happened to him? I couldn't help but ask, the tears now threatening to fall.

Why the fuck, when all his friends are taking their kids to after-school activities, fixing car seats in the back of cars, accompanying their partners to labour wards, having their newborns placed in their arms, getting up at 3.00am for night feeds and gradually developing under-eye bags worthy of any heroin addict, is my DH still not doing, talking about and sharing in any of this stuff?

What did he do to deserve a life that revolves around gruelling fertility appointments and heart-stopping medical invoices and a crazy depressed wife who can't make long-term plans to do anything because she might get pregnant yet, and won't make short-term plans to do anything because she's reeling from the fact that she's still not pregnant now? How has he drawn such an incredibly short straw?

And the answer, I'm afraid, is me. I am the incredibly short straw in this scenario and if he hadn't pulled me then his life would undoubtedly be very different from how it is now.

I've lost count of the naive idiots who've told me how lucky DH and I are to have been brought closer by this unfortunate bump in the road, while all the time they've been busy bickering, arguing and not having sex with their husbands or boyfriends. They smile and tell me how much stronger we must be as a couple, presumably because they can see for themselves that the situation has not quite killed us yet.

If these people must know, our partnership *is* stronger as a result of this nightmare. But I have absolutely no idea how to be a good enough wife to compensate for the children I might never provide. And although we may be stronger, we are most definitely not happier, and I think I can speak for the two of us when I say that we would gladly trade in our newly acquired strength for a happier, less weathered and perhaps altogether weaker relationship.

1.30pm

I've just spent an hour on the phone to my friend Jane and, in between her yelling at her three toddlers to stop trying to poke each other's eyes out with lightsabres, we came to the conclusion that we must arrange to see each other again. She doesn't know when she'll ever find a babysitter deranged enough to take on her brood, and I don't know what I'll feel like doing, or when I'm likely to feel like doing it, but we both agreed that we absolutely must do something and that whatever it is we definitely and absolutely have to do it soon.

I sighed a heavy sigh as I ended the call, and wished that my life, and my feelings towards everyone with children, could just be a little more straightforward.

'You should take up drawing again,' DH informed me a little while later, as I sat eating my croissant and drinking my decaf coffee beside him.

'Why?' I asked him. 'I was never particularly good at it anyway.'

'You were good enough,' he replied, 'and it would be nice for you to have a hobby again.'

'No,' I told him. We were not going to do this today. We were not going to put together some pitiful plan involving crocheting and cake decorating, line dancing and life drawing, hoping that the mind-numbing amalgamation of it all would somehow make us forget how empty our lives really are.

And then I told DH what I really need him to do right now: stop being so bloody solution-focused and just accept our situation for the fucking disaster we both know it is.

7.30pm

Another six toilet trips safely survived. But there is still such a huge expanse of time – around thirty-six long, drawn-out hours, to be precise – in which things could go horribly wrong.

The question now is what will we do if it's bad news once again? Will we honour our earlier agreement that we'd call it quits after three cycles? Or will we succumb to the temptation of 'just one more try' like so many couples who have travelled this road before us?

I've come across several Tarantino women on the forum who, even hours after the discovery of a failed treatment, will defiantly declare: 'I'm never giving up. I refuse to be beaten by this thing.' The war on infertility, they insist, will continue to be fought until it either kills them or they succeed.

I admire their determination, I have to admit, but I don't think I can adopt this standpoint myself.

Ultimately, although our personal limits will vary, there surely must come a time when every one of us is forced to accept defeat. It might be because our partners tell us enough is enough, our bank managers tell us they won't loan us a penny more for this lost cause, or our bodies eventually hit the wall of menopause and dictate that we simply can't try any longer.

It can be hard to recognise when you've reached the end, when natural human instinct will always drive us on, convince us that the surest way to succeed in anything is to try just one last time.

I remember a few years ago, when DH and I first stepped up to this challenge, it felt as though we'd crossed the threshold into a Las Vegas casino, clutching a tight wad of money – the entire contents of everything we'd begged, borrowed and saved – with which to make our fortune.

Now that we're inside the casino, it feels almost impossible to walk away when the chips are still down, when we've lost everything we had to start with, we can't remember how long it is since we last stepped outside, and we'll never know whether our lucky break was almost in our reach.

The longer we've stayed in the casino and the deeper into our final wad of money we've sunk, the more I've started to believe that there is little else to live for if we can't now walk out victorious. And the longer we stay, the more this belief becomes a reality, because we've wreaked so much damage and been absent for so long in the real world that there really is little semblance of our 'real' lives to which we can return.

But for some reason, I, just like the rest of my Tarantino buddies, seem to applaud the never-giving-up approach. When people *do* give up and admit that, as devastating as it is, they know they have reached their limit, their retirement from our club is, for some reason, almost impossible to endorse. Perhaps it's because the rest of us can't bear to acknowledge that the final chapter in our own stories might end on a very similar note.

Giving up, in my opinion, is never easy to do. And it's so hard to decide whether the fear of another failed cycle is preventing us from meeting the baby that is so nearly in view, or whether the fear of never having a baby is forcing us to keep trying things that are both destructive and destined never to work. Probably the hardest thing to accept is that we'll never know for sure.

What I do know for sure is that it will be better for me to make the decision to give up for myself, to effectively walk away while there are still a few cards left on our table.

I choose this every time over the seventeenth review meeting, where Dr Rangan, or his equivalent in whichever clinic we have resorted to, shakes his head, places his hand gently on top of mine and tells me, for the love of God, that we *have* to call it a day – because *he* can't actually take any more.

12.05am

Lying on the bed tonight, DH convinced me that now is the time; time to draw up the plan I've been dreading and to figure out what we're going to do if our official test date in two days' time doesn't bring us the result we want.

For starters, we've both decided that we're going to embrace exercise in a way we've never embraced it before. In fact, I'm going to go one step further than that; I'm going to get ripped. And not like the time I ripped a tendon doing an ambitious yoga posture after our first failed cycle; this time I'm going to acquire the sort of abdominals from which one could bounce a cow.

We've acknowledged that money does not equal happiness, but we've also decided that we'd like to pursue the sort of jobs that will enable us to earn an obscene amount of the stuff.

When this has been accomplished, we will then buy a beautiful house in the country – and a stunning, sea-view penthouse apartment in Spain, Italy or maybe the south of France, which we will visit three times a year. No, six times. At least.

Whilst in Spain, Italy or the south of France, we will spend our time becoming fluent in our second language and also proficient at playing a musical instrument. A proper one, of course, like the guitar or the violin. For fun, we'll learn to surf, which will also give me ample opportunity to acquire a sickening, year-round tan.

Importantly, in whatever spare time we might have, we'll also take up some form of charitable activity; one that isn't too time-consuming and doesn't require us to roll up our sleeves too far, but does prevent other people from making disparaging remarks about our fabulous lifestyle. This way, people can admire us to our faces, but hate us with a seething, barely containable jealousy the minute our backs are turned.

DH and I have tonight visualised ourselves living this lifestyle: lounging in hammocks on the balcony of our holiday apartment, looking impossibly ripped and tanned, strumming our guitars and pausing only to sip on a cocktail and stroke our surfboards.

If we look past a five-year plan, there are inevitable niggling questions that pop up, of course, such as: what will happen when our sickening year-round tans have turned us into a pair of leathery orange suitcases, our hands are too gnarled to strum the guitar and our knees are too knackered to surf? And to whom will we leave our glittering cross-European property empire?

But who cares about ten- or twenty-year plans? As a five- year draft, what we have come up with is not too depressing.

Well, that was what we'd agreed, but then DH decided to quite innocently ask a question…and the goodwill and laughter that had filled our flat this evening evaporated in an instant.

'How're the guys?' was the question he asked me, nodding towards my belly as I stood by the bathroom mirror removing the day's makeup with a wad of cotton wool.

'I wish I knew,' I whispered.

It wasn't what he wanted to hear; he wanted me to tell him that they're doing just fine, that after all our hard work and his hard-earned money to get them here, my body is, *of course*, doing all it can to uphold its end of the bargain. But I can't make these sorts of promises, and he should know that by now.

I hate it when he asks about Kenneth and Donaghy. It makes me feel so incredibly guilty when I'm forced to admit that my duplicitous body might very well have dispatched of our precious babies for the third time in a row.

I can't blame him for wanting to communicate with them and spur them on, and I know *I've* been talking to the little fellas at regular intervals throughout the day. But as soon as I witnessed DH doing it, the whole thing suddenly felt like such a ridiculous sham – and I knew that I was the one propelling it.

I feel as though I've been deliberately lying to him for the last two weeks, and as though I'm pulling the wool over his eyes tonight, when I know that as he rubs my belly he's saying goodnight to nothing more exciting than the semi-digested bowl of bran flakes I've just eaten as a guilt-free midnight snack.

'It'll be okay if it's bad news,' he said, gently rubbing my belly as we lay side by side in the dark. 'I can find a way to be happy – even if it is just the two of us, you know.'

'Well, I can't,' I replied, without hesitation.

He laughed and asked me to explain exactly what I was saying; whether I seriously meant that he couldn't be enough for me on his own.

I stared through the darkness towards the ceiling and told him, unflinchingly, that of course he could never begin to compensate for the baby I may now never know.

I'm not sure where the words came from, but I know they were not what I'd wanted to say.

What I wanted to somehow articulate is that I don't want to hear him tolerating this second-rate life. I wanted to scream at him

– or at someone – that this world is currently stuffed to the rafters with crummy, useless and undeserving fathers, and here he is, so cut out for the job, and I can't bear to watch him just stand there and shrug and accept that he'll never get the chance.

But I couldn't find the words or even the will to say any of those things.

And now, as I lie in the dark, alone and in the knowledge that I've just destroyed the one constant I did have in my future, I've decided, here and now, to broaden the criteria for the happy ending I desire.

In two days' time, I just want to awaken, either to the discovery of a positive pregnancy test, or to the discovery that I suddenly and inexplicably no longer want a baby.

Imagine the joy of a positive pregnancy test after all this time! And then imagine the liberation of realising that it doesn't matter anymore; that I am alive and healthy, that tomorrow is the first day of the rest of my life, and that I can take this life and do with it exactly as I please.

Yes! There are two possible ways to break free from this nightmare, two possible ways to start smiling and living my life again. And, hand on my heart, from this point forward I just want the universe to know that I no longer have even a first choice.

I will leave it to the hand of fate, I will stop wishing and hoping and pleading, and I will gladly take either one.

Day Fourteen – Monday 13th February

And They'll Tell You Hope Dies Last

Symptoms: Extreme nausea, sweaty palms, palpitations, sore boobs, moderate stomach cramps, flatulence and a very dry mouth.

Hours remaining: 24

Waking hours remaining: 24 (no sense in kidding myself now; there'll be no sleep tonight)

Predicted odds on this working: 0.00000001/10

6.10am

It comes as no surprise to discover that sleep – and general mental functioning – are elusive to a woman who is charging to the toilet every five minutes to check the contents of her knickers.

Each half-hourly toilet victory now feels monumental, and at the same time completely inconsequential. There must be at least another ten toilet trips to survive before the big event and, even if I outlast all ten of them, I must still overcome the titanic hurdle of the home pregnancy test before we can call this a success.

Amidst staring robotically at the TV's morning news coverage, I've been trying to present myself with a mental conveyor belt of all the comforting things I get to indulge in once this negative pregnancy test is out of the way.

To start, I'm going to have a volcanically hot bath, of previously forbidden, embryo-boiling temperatures, swiftly followed by a gallon of coffee, a giant chocolate bar and a bottle of the finest red wine I can afford (whatever is on special offer at the local garage, then).

In terms of slightly longer-term plans, I don't have anything much different from what I came up with after our second cycle, which is distressing to say the least, since the requirement for solid, longer-term plans is so much more urgent this time around.

We do have our 'seize the day' five-year plan that we mapped out in bed last night, of course, but – not wanting to underplay the gratification that would accompany having abdominals from which one could bounce a cow – on reflection I'm not convinced it contains anything of lifelong significance just yet.

11.15am

The flat feels very empty without DH here, now that I've been left with only my own indelible words about his 'not being enough' ringing in my head.

For the last hour I've been sat by the window, staring down at the scurrying people on the street, eagerly getting on with their frenetic Monday morning schedules. And I've been ruminating on my own frenetic schedule, my very private mission, my solitary five-year battle that I have waged inside this tiny London flat, unbeknownst to the bustling world outside.

It seems that this uncontrollable desire to have a baby has torn through my life like a tsunami, leaving little but a ghost town in its wake. Even my husband now appears as a faint, distant silhouette, barely discernible amidst the wreckage that lies all around.

I find myself today standing alone in the last remaining watchtower, surveying the hanging tatters of a life that lie in every direction and as far as the eye can see. And although I'm aware that I continue to wake up each morning, and my blood still runs through my veins, I couldn't say that I feel in any way alive.

Whatever happens from here on in, I know now that it is time for me to descend from this watchtower, to pick through the ruins outside and to salvage all the elements that I'll need to rebuild a life. It will take time to build something stable, functional and pretty enough for other people to want to come and visit again. But it is not beyond my means. I just need to look around me at people the world over; human beings are rolling up their sleeves to embark upon this kind of 'reconstruction after tragedy' project every single day.

But I can't, and I don't want to, start this project alone. I need my companion and my friend; I need my 'DH' at my side.

Maybe it is time for our roles to be reversed and for me to lead the way; to place my hands firmly on his shoulders, look him squarely in the eye and assure him that everything is going to be okay. It may not suit my mood and it may not be anywhere close to what I believe, but I think now could be the time for me to return his five-year-long favour and simply start lying for the sake of the person I love.

2.10pm

In amongst the dreaded but necessary toilet visits, I've spent the last couple of hours emailing Goldilocks, who apparently lives in a small town just north of Stockholm. Mostly, I've been trying to reassure her that the five negative pregnancy tests she's taken *might* still be wrong. I wouldn't have patronised her with these hollow words of comfort if she hadn't made it clear that she has no desire just yet to face the truth.

Goldilocks might be in a remote Swedish town around nine hundred miles away from me, but this woman's anguish has transcended the distance that lies between us and this afternoon is palpable within the four walls of my home.

I've met the grim reaper of embryos whom Goldilocks so understandably fears. He's a bitter acquaintance of mine, and has chosen to darken my doorstep on two separate nights before now. Today, once again, I can feel his nefarious presence closing in, and I, like Goldilocks, feel in no rush whatsoever to let him cross the threshold and sweep back in here into our lives.

It is strange and out of character, but for some reason Goldilocks's negative test results have brought me not a scrap of consolation today. Six months ago they would have brought me an unpleasant kind of reassurance, perhaps proving that I was not alone in my misfortune. I might even have received the news of these results with a shameful flicker of relief, illogically hoping that if another woman's journey had just been rounded off with the much-feared BFN, then maybe, just maybe, there would be an extra space for my name on the list of BFPs.

Today, however, Goldilocks's news has only expanded the vacuum within my heart. Have I finally accepted that we're each in this race alone, that the events happening to other people can never have any real influence over the path our lives will take? Or have I merely come to realise that I don't want this particular brand of misery to attract the company of others any longer?

4.30pm

I have run out of things to tidy, file away and rearrange and I've occupied the rest of the afternoon by emailing Nat, chatting on the phone to my mum, forcing down half an omelette and watching five back-to-back episodes of *Game of Thrones* (season 3).

And I doubt I could recall a single second of any of it.

I shouldn't put it off any longer. I need to tell DH that I didn't mean it when I said that I'd gladly trade him in for a baby. What I meant to say is that I want to have a baby *with* him, *because* of him, even. I need to tell him that, although he may not be able to fulfil my need to be a mother (no matter how untidy he may be) and in all honesty he may never quite fill the void left by infertility, he will come far closer to filling it than any other human ever could.

I need to tell him that, as much as I'm determined to sometimes, I couldn't ever bring myself to hate my life entirely while he plays such a starring role within it.

I need to tell him that there *is* hope for the two of us, with or without a baby.

And I need to tell him that I haven't ever told him any of this before because, in my strange, superstitious way, I haven't wanted to stand here and admit that I'll find a way to cope whatever happens. I haven't wanted to risk giving the universe the choice, and so I've told it in no uncertain terms that I could never be strong enough to bear this cross forever.

Ultimately, I need to do the unthinkable and tell DH that I was wrong and he was right – about pretty much everything.

5.30pm

Oh, how I wish I had a crystal ball to see into our future. Maybe then I could see our adopted children, who are being conceived somewhere in the world this very afternoon, coming into our lives on a bright summer's day in a few years' time. Or maybe I could leap ahead to December 2050, and watch as a steady stream of well-rounded adults, whom DH and I have fostered to maturity over the course of our colourful lives, come to our door to wish us a merry Christmas.

Or perhaps I could drop in on myself a couple of weeks after my fortieth birthday, find myself perched on the edge of a toilet seat, pregnancy test stick clutched in my trembling hand, praying with every fibre of my being that the universe wasn't going to finally grant me a pass into motherhood, when having a baby would only serve to ruin the extraordinary life I'd so painstakingly built in its place.

What a wonderfully and ironically poetic ending to this journey that might be.

7.15pm

I've spent far too much time today scouring the pages of the Internet for stories of women who, just like me, felt convinced beyond all doubt that their treatments had failed, when in fact they had been pregnant all along.

I've found a couple of stories from women who swear you could have knocked them down with a feather when their test sticks displayed a positive rather than a negative result; women whose stories sound more than a little familiar, because I'm pretty sure I was dredging them up at around this time in my last cycle. And the one before that, too.

I'm 99.999999999 per cent certain that there are no feathers waiting to waft down from the skies and knock me off my feet tomorrow morning, but hope, as they say, is notoriously last to die.

Even when you believe every last trace of it has vanished for good, sure enough if you look more closely, a shred of it will remain, doggedly clinging on until you've reached a point that you're certain is several miles further on from the bitter end.

I want to command this final shred to curl up and die like all the other shreds that have gradually peeled away and withered in the earlier days of this two-week wait.

Years ago, I might have believed that this final shred of hope will cling on only until the negative pregnancy test is staring me in the face – but I know better than to believe that now.

I know this last, stubborn, weather-beaten strand of mental stamina will already be bracing itself for another negative result and will have a well-rehearsed speech prepared, oiled and ready to roll out should the need arise.

I will say that this is it, we have reached the end, we can officially do no more. And, right on cue, the shred of hope will sidle in, scrape my head off the floor, point to the horizon and whisper in my ear that it isn't over yet. There are *always* stories of women who have several unsuccessful rounds of IVF and then get pregnant naturally. I am not menopausal yet, you know, and there is still next month, and the month after that. Not to mention the month after that. It *could* still happen.

It must go without saying that I detest this shred of hope. It slays me in a uniquely relentless way that despair could never attempt to match. You know where you are with despair, and invariably that's in bed with the duvet up over your head, on the sofa with a greyhound and a cold tin of baked beans in your lap, or in a ramshackle watering hole at the end of a bottle of gin.

The final shred of hope will show no such mercy. Exhausting son of a bitch that it is, it will demand that I pull myself together. Whatever happens, it will simply tell me to hang on in there, to stack the deck and to keep on playing in the certainty that it's simply not possible for every hand in life to be this much of a bust.

I'm starting to worry there may be no escape from this instinctive human need to focus on the bright side of life. Back when we were teenagers, I remember Jane, Nat and I used to stay up late at weekends watching horror films and screaming at the characters on the screen, imploring them to kill themselves quickly before the chainsaw-wielding psychopath could inflict a gruesome ending upon them.

'I'd knock myself out! I'd shoot myself in the head!' we all yelled at the screen.

But if the last five years have taught me anything, it's that

I wouldn't knock myself out or shoot myself in the head. Because the shred of hope would be there, accompanying me until the very end, reassuring me that, as unlikely as it seemed, things *could* still turn around. There was still a chance that the chainsaw-wielding psychopath might suffer a timely cardiac arrest, or trip on a cable and accidentally quarter himself right before my head was about to be sawn off.

And if the shred of hope would stand by me while the psychopath wielded his chainsaw above my head, then I know it will be fearless enough to stick with me through whatever happens tomorrow morning.

8.30pm

I have sent a series of words to DH, together with a photo of the two of us, windswept but smiling, taken on the top deck of a ferry to France, right after he proposed six years ago. The words I have written are not quite right and are nowhere close to enough – but then an apology of this magnitude must either start somewhere or else forever be left unsaid.

11.30pm

So, this is it, then. Tomorrow is D-day. The toilet-terrors threatened by this day have again been averted, but this confirms nothing other than the fact that we are still in with a chance. I can't help but play out the final dramatic scene of this two-week wait in my head, and I'm sure that DH is doing exactly the same, even though he's lying beside me in bed pretending to be watching something mildly entertaining on his laptop.

Through a long-lens camera and with the sound turned to mute, a film taken of the first minute or so of tomorrow morning would probably look pretty much the same in either of the two endings that have pre-emptively been shot: two sleep-starved people standing in their pyjamas in a harshly lit bathroom, clinging to each other as though an earthquake is erupting beneath their feet.

Carry on watching for a few moments, and the differences will be revealed: the two figures slowly slumping to the ground, heads bowed – or throwing their heads back to the sky, jumping up and down and spinning each other round the room in wild abandon.

There is no middle ground and no consolation prize in this game. It is do or die; the nosedive to rock bottom or the rocket launch to cloud nine.

I wonder which two-minute film we'll be enacting tomorrow morning. I really would like to try the happy ending this time.

As soon as he walked through the door tonight, DH locked me in a wordless hug and the two of us stood and cried for what could have been either ten minutes or several hours.

I don't deserve him, that much is certain, but I am eternally grateful that he is still here and that he is willing to put up with me for a while longer at least.

I can't even imagine how wonderful it would feel if things genuinely turned out to be okay.

How I'd love to see two lines on one of those wretched little sticks.

How I'd love to see tears of happiness in DH's eyes and feel them in my own.

How I'd love to go for a walk into town, hand in hand, smiling uncontrollably whenever we catch each other's eye, because we're thinking about the brand-new secret person-in-the-making about whom only the two of us know.

How I'd love to feel fat and uncomfortable and as sick as a dog.

How I'd love to argue over names and the colour of the

nursery, and daydream about what our son or daughter would be like: whose kind of hair, whose sense of humour, whose approach to life?

How I'd love to fear stretch marks and piles and episiotomies and lie awake at night wondering how on earth we'll cope with the enormity of all our new responsibilities and what the fuck we've gone and done.

'So, what time shall I set the alarm for tomorrow morning, then?' DH joked before turning out the light on his bedside table.

I think we both know we'll be up with the sparrows tomorrow morning – if, that is, we ever manage to fall asleep tonight.

The test sticks have been retrieved from their hiding place in the spare room and are now sitting on the edge of the bathtub waiting for their moment of glory in a few hours' time. And I'm lying here, heart racing, simultaneously hoping that tomorrow morning hurries up and that it never gets here at all.

Unavoidably, however, it *will* get here, and when it does and I'm holding in my quivering hand one of those stupid plastic sticks, I hope I manage to spare a thought for all the other women across the world whose personal storylines will also have brought them, at that exact moment in time, to the very edge of their toilet seats, a small plastic stick clutched inside their own sweating palms.

Between us, we'll reside in every location, from the populated cities of Tokyo, London and Mumbai, to the rugged landscapes of the Himalayas and Mount Cameroon. We will belong to all age groups, demographics, backgrounds and beliefs.

Amongst us will be the ones who are dreading a positive result: teenagers who forgot to use a condom, girls whose boyfriends are complete wastes of space, women in their twenties who had a barely recollected one-night stand, women who've been the victims of rape, and exhausted mothers who already have four children under the age of five.

And then there will be the other women, women who have, like me, been trying to get pregnant for as long as they can remember; women who are facing what could be their last ever chance of one day hearing the word 'Mum'.

If there were a room anywhere in the world big enough to hold us all under one roof, there would right now be a deafening cacophony; fifty languages combining to voice one of two desperate pleas, offered up to a god or gods whom we may or may not have believed in prior to this pivotal moment in our lives.

What a terrible shame it is that all of our plastic sticks can't be collected in a giant pot and redistributed according to our needs.

In the aftermath of tomorrow's results, I guess we'll all find a way to move on with our lives. Win or lose, tomorrow's test will simply be chalked down as yet another small entry in our long and chaotic life stories.

And I know I can rest assured that, win or lose, there will be bigger days to come. Days that involve giving birth to our babies in labour wards in nine months' time, or maybe, for some of us, something…else. Something I couldn't begin to imagine tonight, but something that I have to believe will amount to a whole lot more than all the negative pregnancy tests I've held in my hand over the last five years.

I've just bid Goldilocks and my other Tarantino buddies farewell and a final good luck for tomorrow morning, and they have each returned their good wishes to me.

I can't speak on behalf of the others, of course, but I think that maybe this time when I wished them all good luck, I might have even meant it. For once, I might genuinely be wishing upon them the result that they are praying for themselves, instead of wishing upon them only the same result that's waiting in store for me.

Could it be that the bilious alter-ego within is starting to loosen her grip on me at last?

For a long time I feared that she would surely outlive me, that I would wither and she would be the one to take the body we share through to a bitter and twisted old age.

But perhaps, in the end and against all the odds, this arduous journey might just prove the death of her before it can prove the death of me.

When I think of all the women who'll be sharing tomorrow's D-day with me, all I can do is to wish them all someone in their lives who'll pull them through no matter what the outcome. Someone like DH, who's lying next to me right now and who has just started snoring like he hasn't a care in the world (men: you've got to love them).

As for me, how I wish I had something life-affirming and poignant to say; some sort of powerful epiphany to share about not wasting any more of my precious time on this earth, not wishing for anything too prescriptive in this life and instead gratefully embracing the unexpected twists and turns of our existence and accepting happiness in whatever form it may take.

But I would be the worst kind of liar if I were to spin anyone that kind of a line tonight.

The truth is that there are four words that pull me from my sleep each morning, four words I whisper into my pillow each night, and four words that play on a loop in my brain for every minute and every second that pass in between.

I want a baby. I want a baby. I. Want. A. Baby.

This haunting biological imperative has taken a hold of my heart, of my head, and of my soul – and I do not believe that it will ever now let me go.

Acknowledgements

With huge thanks to my much-missed dad (the first person to read an early draft of this book, and my inspiration for writing it); my mum for always being there; my DH for keeping the laughter alive; and my wonderful family and friends, both real and virtual – you know who you are and I hope you know how lucky I feel to have you in my life.